2023 KETO LOW-CARB DIET GUIDE

NEW UPDATES FOR BEGINNERS AND KETOGENIC BURNOUTS TO RESET, GET MOTIVATED AND MAXIMIZE WEIGHT LOSSNEW UPDATES FOR BEGINNERS AND KETOGENIC BURNOUTS TO RESET, GET MOTIVATED AND MAXIMIZE WEIGHT LOSS

TAYLOR NEAL

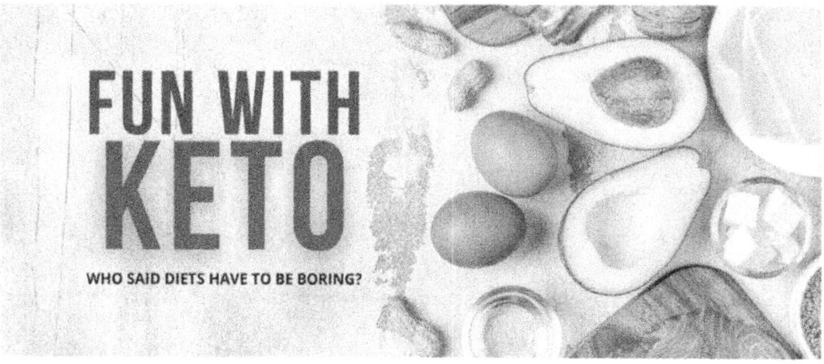

Find your tribe at **FUN WITH KETO!** A positive community focused on keeping your diet fun as you pursue a lifestyle change with the ketogenic diet. Here you will find sharing of personal success stories, keto hacks, the latest diet updates, tips, new ideas, and delicious quick-prep recipes shared by our moderators and members. Keto is more fun when you surround yourself with community:

SCAN ME

https://www.facebook.com/groups/funwithketo

CONTENTS

Introduction vii

1. The Ups and Downs of Dieting 1
2. Keto Updates and Innovations 6
3. The Quick Start Guide to Kickstart You Into Ketosis 31
4. Nutrition 44
5. Health and Fitness With Keto 86
6. Staying On Track and Keeping Yourself Accountable 94
7. Bounce Back Stronger 105
8. Debunking Myths and Fixing Common Mistakes 135
9. Stay Motivated With Keto Success Stories 154

Afterword 171
References 173

INTRODUCTION

Like so many other people, I felt the need to lose weight in order to regain control over my life and health again. However, every diet that I tried got me nowhere but frustrated with the lack of movement on the scale. Plus, I was miserable from the dietary restrictions, and felt like I was depriving myself of sustenance and still feeling hungry throughout the day. My body was fighting my effort and hard work, and I didn't know what to try next. Then, I learned about the ketogenic diet, and my life started to transform before my very eyes.

I lost 40 pounds in the initial few months, and while I was happy with the progress, a burnout surely followed. I wasn't creative with my meals and made mistakes early on that caused me to plateau. I attempted to liven up my meals with plant-based alternatives, like almond flour, almond milk, and protein powders, and once again, I was back on track. Soon after the addition to these plant-based alternatives, my body began to turn on me. I suffered from a severe asthma attack that left me hospitalized, where I found out that I am deathly allergic to nuts. The alternatives that I had been putting into my body nearly killed me, and this realization stalled my progress.

After my near-death discovery, I decided to take a small break from the keto diet while I recovered. Within no time, I had gained back 15 of the original 40 pounds that I had lost, and I decided to try keto again. However, my body started to fight back once again, so I started to do some research on the ketogenic diet. Through my research, I found that there are other ways that I could live a ketogenic lifestyle without endangering my life due to my allergy. I found that there are alternative keto plans, like the standard, targeted, high-protein, and vegan plans.

I slowly started to recover and have since lost those regained pounds and more. I became passionate about living a ketogenic lifestyle, and I thought to myself, *What do I do with all this research and knowl-*

edge about keto that I have learned? Surely there are people out there that don't know its benefits or even how it works. That's what made me decide to write this book. Not only do I want the people beginning in their keto journey to be well informed about how the ketosis process works, but I want the people who have been on keto for years to be updated on the information that has come out since they started. Life can become hectic and keeping up with all of the new information and recipes can seem like just another task for a busy day. So putting all of the information in one place may take the edge off, make your life a little easier, inspire you to restart and liven up your diet, and increase your passion for a ketogenic lifestyle.

1

THE UPS AND DOWNS OF DIETING

So many people start a new diet with a feeling of hopefulness for a new beginning. They change everything about their lifestyle: the way that they eat, how much they eat, and how often or intensely they work out. However, after not seeing the progress that they assumed they would have in a short amount of time, or hitting their first plateau, they are quick to give up and try something else.

While some people manage to lose weight and meet their goal, they slowly go back to the way that they were living before they started their weight-loss journey. They stop counting their calories, increase their runs through the drive-thru, and lose the motivation to get up early in the morning to work out.

To their dismay, they regain all of the weight that they worked so hard to lose and possibly some extra pounds.

SO MANY RESOURCES, SO LITTLE TIME

All day, every day, all we hear about is dieting or the newest trends to get that hourglass shape that we always wanted. Every month, a new diet book comes out, and the grocery store checkout lane is littered with health magazines. You turn on the television and every other commercial is for new diet pills or the newest innovation in weight loss. With so much information thrown at you throughout the day, how could you simply know the truth about dieting? How do you know what diets are scientifically proven to work and which ones are just a new trend in the never-ending cycle of fad diets? It's no wonder that there are so many people switching from diet to diet until they find one that actually works and makes them feel better without feeling malnourished and deprived of their joy.

TRY, FAIL, GET BACK UP AGAIN

Motivation and resilience are a requirement when it comes to losing weight. As I stated before, so many people grow frustrated when they aren't dropping the pounds as quickly as they thought they would, or their neighbor did by using the same exact method. They grow tired of giving up the food that they love without having anything to show for it. Sometimes, they slip up and have food on their 'banned' list during a night out with friends. Then, they are overcome with shame or self-loathing because of their lack of self-control, and instead of getting back on track, they just keep going with their unhealthy eating habits.

Eating food that isn't generally on your diet on occasion will happen. Life was meant to be enjoyed, within reason of course. Making a mistake or overindulging because you already ate something you weren't supposed to doesn't mean that you just as easily get back on track the next morning. Remembering to set realistic goals and trying not to compare yourself to others' weight-loss success will keep you from getting discouraged with your own progress. Everybody loses weight differently, and we tend to forget that there are many factors that contribute to why some people lose weight faster than others. Hormones, age, body type, and genetics are just a few examples of these factors.

PIECING TOGETHER A WORKING PUZZLE

Finding what works for you during this journey is the most important aspect of dieting. It is a trial-and-error basis, as long as the trial is long enough to properly judge whether the diet is actually working for you and making you feel happier, healthier, and more fulfilled. There are, on some occasions, medical reasons why you aren't losing weight. Some people, like me, may have an allergy to certain alternative supplements that they are using in their healthier eating habits. Some people may have a slower metabolism due to an undiagnosed thyroid disorder. If you have tried different diets without any success, you may need to make an appointment with your family doctor and see what is going on. After some blood work, your doctor may be able to point you in the right direction of what changes you could make in your eating habits that will help you get to your goal weight.

WINNING AT ANY AGE

For the people who aren't quite 20-years-old anymore, they may notice that they have had a major decline in their metabolism as they get older. As we age, we lose our muscle mass, go through hormonal changes, our stress level increases, and our activity level slows down. Women normally start the stage of menopause at the age of 45, and that decrease in their estrogen levels can bring on the extra pounds around the waistline. Men's testosterone levels start to drop around the age of 40. Since testosterone helps with how the fat is distributed, muscle mass, and strength, men's ability to burn calories the way that they did when they were younger is much more difficult.

There are also issues with the involuntary disintegration of your muscle mass and fatty tissue taking over the muscle composition as they age. However, even if the odds are stacked against you, that doesn't mean that you can't lose weight. Everyone has a certain barrier that they are afraid will hold them back when it comes to weight loss, but as long as you are motivated and consistent in your attempts, there should be no reason why you can't meet your goal.

2

KETO UPDATES AND INNOVATIONS

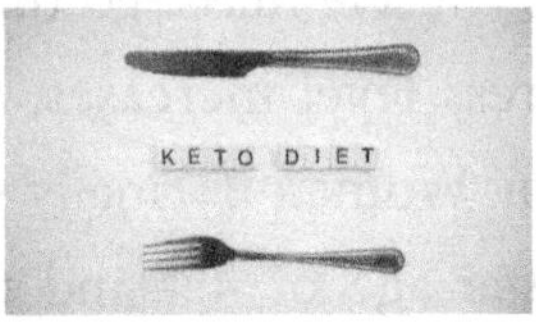

A BRIEF HISTORY OF THE KETO DIET

The ketogenic diet has grown in popularity in the last decade, but many people would be surprised of its complete history and how it wasn't even thought about until a nation-wide news channel ran a report in 1994 that brought it back into the media's eye. The keto diet has been used since the 1920s as a way to decrease the occurrence of seizures in pediatric epileptic patients, but the research for the change in diet started in France in 1911 until it was proven to show improvement in patients. Before that time, the only way that doctors knew about decreasing the severity and how often the seizures occurred was by fasting. While the results were impressive, with it benefiting 50% of adults and 90% of pediatric patients, these results were proven as only a temporary cure and the illness would return soon after.

Doctors conducted more research by modifying diets, mostly focused on cutting out sugars and starchy foods. Dr. Wilder, a physician at the Mayo Clinic, noticed that a handful of his patients showed more progress when their sugar intake was lowered rather than the traditional approach, especially when they were following a high-fat, low-carb diet. By mimicking how fasting changes a patient's metabolism, Dr. Wilder came up with the first guidelines of a ketogenic diet.

The keto diet worked well for epileptics because the low amount of sugar and glucose intake and high amount of healthy fats consumed altered the brain's ability to become over-excited, and lowered the chances of the brain to generate seizures. The decreasing occurrence of seizures made it possible for epileptics to stop taking their anti-seizure medications, but doctors started to notice their patient's weight loss as a result of the diet. Dr. Peterman, another physician at the Mayo Clinic, took Dr.

Wilder's guidelines and created the standard keto diet that is still being used today.

Without the dedication that doctors and researchers put forth in helping epileptic patients, the world would not have the ketogenic diet. People that have struggled to lose weight for years on end without any success, or have had difficulties managing their diabetes and blood sugar would feel hopeless. There are medical breakthroughs every day, whether it's for diseases, diets, or research studies. The only way to figure out what makes people happier and healthier are tested methods over a long amount of time and seeing how it affects their lives.

Multiple studies have found that the keto diet is more effective when it comes to weight loss than just a low-fat, low-calorie diet. One study stated that a ketogenic diet helped people lose more than two times the amount of weight than other restrictive diets (Brehm et al., 2003). It is also successful in helping people feel full for a longer time throughout the day, cutting down on how much they can eat and how often they feel hungry.

History may be boring to a few, but if we don't acknowledge how far that the ketogenic diet has come, how much it has changed, and it has helped others, then we won't be able to appreciate what it could do for future generations. The last thing that humans want is for their children, grandchildren, or even great-grandchildren to suffer the pain that they felt because they were overweight, especially when there are simple changes that can be made in their diet to stay healthy.

WHAT IS KETO EXACTLY AND HOW DOES IT WORK?

Everyone remembers when the Atkins diet became extremely popular in the late 1990s. The keto and Atkins diet are similar due to the fact that they both restrict the amount of carbohydrates you can eat per day. However, keto is considered a high-fat, medium-protein, low-carb diet, whereas Atkins limits the amount of fats you can consume.

When you drastically decrease the amount of your carb intake and replace the carbs with healthy fats, your body goes through a different metabolic state known as ketosis. A body in ketosis will have lower insulin and blood sugar levels and will rely on the fatty foods that you eat for its energy source rather than relying on the sugar found in carbohydrates.

There are different versions of keto diet plans: standard, targeted, cyclical, and high protein. The standard ketogenic diet consists of 70% fat, 20% protein, and about 10% carbs rationed throughout the day. The targeted ketogenic diet allows you to add carbs to your diet revolving around your workout schedule. The cyclical ketogenic diet consists of five days of strict low-carb intake, followed by two days of eating food high in carbs. The high-protein ketogenic diet follows the same guidelines as the standard version but adds more protein into the percentages. The ratio for the high-protein version is 65% fats, 35% proteins, and 5% carbs.

OTHER BENEFITS YOU CAN GAIN FROM A KETOGENIC LIFESTYLE

There are so many other benefits to the keto diet besides losing weight. A high-fat, low-carb diet leads to losing fat around your midsection. Not all body fat is considered to be the same, and losing belly fat lowers risk of inflammation, diabetes, and insulin resistance. The drastic drop in triglycerides decreases the risk of developing heart disease, a risk that consuming large quantities of carbohydrates plays a major part in.

A ketogenic diet increases your HDL cholesterol, also known as the 'good cholesterol.' The goal is to have your HDL cholesterol higher than your LDL cholesterol, thereby lowering your chances of heart problems or cardiac events in the future. Restricting your carb intake can reduce your blood sugar and your insulin levels, making diabetes management much easier to control. It also lowers your blood pressure, decreasing the chances for multiple diseases, including stroke, kidney disease, and heart failure. The keto diet is even helpful in improving acne, sleep quality, and PCOS symptoms.

Then there are all of the mental health benefits that you gain from being on the keto diet. Obviously, as you lose weight, you will gain confidence and be in a better mood, but the mental health aspect goes much further than that. Many psychologists have recommended that people with mental illnesses or disorders, such as bipolar disorders 1 and 2, autism spectrum disorder, depression, ADHD, anxiety, and PTSD try going on a ketogenic, or at least a low-carb diet. The reason for this recommendation is that a ketogenic diet stabilizes stress hormones, reduces brain inflammation, helps with appetite, rebalance neurotransmitters, and can keep the side effect of weight gain caused by most psychiatric medications at bay. By reducing the amount of processed food that someone with a mental illness or disorder consumes, you could also reduce how often and how severe their symptoms occur (Ede, 2019).

KETOSIS 101

Many of the body's cells rely on sugar for fuel, and the limited access to glucose in the bloodstream makes the body change its fuel source to fat. A low-carb diet lowers the insulin in your body and fatty acids that are being stored in your body storage are released. Most of the fatty acids move to the liver, where they become oxidized and are transformed into ketones. The ketones allow you to lose weight quickly because it decreases the sugar and water that are being stored in the body. The reduction in the water and glycogen in your body suppresses your appetite, allowing you to easily lower your caloric intake. There are some cells in the brain that rely on glucose to function, and the majority of the protein in your diet produces the glucose that your brain needs while in ketosis. Many people confuse ketosis with ketoacidosis, a Type 1 (and on occasion Type 2) diabetes complication that releases a dangerous level of ketones and blood sugars into the bloodstream making the blood acidic.

There are other benefits to getting into ketosis besides weight loss. The reduction in your insulin levels can improve your insulin sensitivity that can contribute to obesity and Type 2 diabetes. Reducing your carb intake lowers your blood triglycerides, HDL cholesterol, and your total cholesterol. The lower levels of these three improve your heart health, and decrease the risk for heart disease. The keto diet is frequently used to reduce epileptic seizures in children, often resulting in the child no longer needing medication. A 2005 study, held at St. Luke's Roosevelt Health Center in New York, found that after 28 days of following a strict keto diet someone with Parkinson's Disease can see a significant improvement in their symptoms (VanItallie et al., 2005).

WHAT FOODS GET YOU INTO KETOSIS?

To get into ketosis, you have to start decreasing your carbohydrates intake to fewer than 50 carbs per day and eventually lower it to fewer than 25 carbs. Of course, the number of carbohydrates that someone can consume to reach ketosis varies, depending on the person. In order to get into ketosis, you have to cut out certain types of foods, including grains, sugary drinks and snacks, processed foods, artificial sweeteners, milk, refined oils, legumes, high-carb and sugary fruits, and potatoes.

Vegetables can be tricky when it comes to which ones are low in carbs, but remember that ones that grow above ground are usually lower in carbohydrates. Veggies that are considered 'root' vegetables, like carrots, can be eaten in moderation. Try sticking to non-starchy vegetables, like leafy greens, zucchini, cucumber, asparagus, and celery.

Some fruits are permitted on the keto diet, if they are eaten in moderation. Avocados are low in carbs and high in fat content and fiber, making them a heart-healthy fruit. A 3.5-ounce serving of avocado is only 1.5 net carbs. Berries, like raspberries, strawberries, and blueberries, are considered to be very low in carbs and calories, and they are high in fiber. A half cup of fresh strawberries is 4.3 net carbs and 45 calories. Using lemons as a sweetener in your iced water can be a great addition because not only does it taste great, but the pectin in lemons can lower blood sugar levels and reduce joint inflammation. A whole lemon only has 4.0 net carbs and is loaded with fiber.

Healthy oils, like olive and avocado oil, are used in most recipes. Coconut oil can be used while on the keto diet but using it too much may raise your LDL cholesterol, also known as the 'bad' cholesterol. These oils also fall into the category of healthy fats on the keto diet, along with nut and seed butters, a variety of nuts (walnuts, almonds, macadamias, etc.), and butter.

There are so many different choices of where to get your protein on keto. Some people prefer a variety of meats, such as beef, poultry, seafood, veal, and venison. You can get protein from other sources like nuts and nut butters. There is protein in eggs and cheese. Plant-based proteins come from tofu and vegan cream cheese or butter.

FOODS TO AVOID

The list of foods to avoid while on the keto diet is shorter than one would believe, but that is because most of the food belongs to the same food groups: sugars, starches, and grains. Grains that include wheat flour, such as breads, oatmeal, and pasta, are very high in carbohydrates and can keep you from getting into ketosis. Vegetables, like corn and carrots, are higher in carbs than the suggested veggies, and can be consumed occasionally. As long as you track the amount that you eat and don't make them a part of your daily meal plan, they won't hinder your progress. However, there are some vegetables that you should avoid at all costs, including (but not limited to):

- yams or sweet potatoes
- potatoes
- beets
- parsnips
- peas

Fruits, besides low-carb berries, are also on the "no-fly zone" list. While fruit has a high fiber content, it also contains large amounts of glucose and carbohydrates. Fruits that you should stay far away from include:

- apples
- mangoes
- grapes and raisins
- bananas

- peaches
- prunes
- dates
- pineapples
- pears
- cranberries (fresh or dried)

Legumes and beans contain large amounts of protein, fiber, and zinc that would be beneficial to other diets; however, the high carb content would only hinder your progress. The list of legumes that are to be avoided include:

- lentils
- lobia
- lima beans
- black beans
- green peas
- baked beans
- kidney beans

MAKING THOSE MACROS AND CALORIES COUNT

With the keto diet, you will constantly hear the word 'macros,' but for someone just starting out, you may be wondering what are macros? The word 'macros' is short for the term macronutrients, and for this diet the three main macros to track are fats, proteins, and carbs. If you are focusing on losing weight, it makes sense to focus on what you are eating and staying on track. Calories are just important to track, but with macro counting, you are able to see where those calories are coming from so you can make the most of your meals.

Keeping track of your macros can help you lose weight quickly. It can also help you maintain your lean muscle mass, while you learn what ratios work for you to keep your body feeling full and satisfied. In the beginning of your keto journey, don't be surprised if your macros may be over your daily allowance and you are still hungry at the end of the day. You will slowly learn how to plan your meals ahead of time when you are tracking so you can stay on track and see the benefits of the diet.

You have two choices when it comes to how you calculate your carb intake on the ketogenic diet: total carbs or net carbs. When calculating your total carbs, you are basically taking the number in the carbohydrates section of a food label for what it is. If a nutrition label says that one serving of peanut butter is 8.0 carbohydrates, then that is what you would count. However, for net carbs you would take the amount of total carbs and subtract the amount of fiber. Staying with the previous example of peanut butter, the total carbs states 8.0 g and the amount of fiber states 2.0 g, meaning that the number of net carbs in one serving of peanut butter is 6.0 g of carbs per serving.

The thought of doing math all day long while you are counting your macros and trying to figure out if you are over your daily allowance may seem like a lot of work. However, using an online tracker website or an app on your phone can help take the stress off of you. You will learn about how these apps work in the next section.

THE NEWEST KETO UPDATES

Life is changing every day and always evolving, and so is the keto diet. New innovations and updates are being made or discovered all the time that will help you lose weight and get over that plateau.

SUPPLEMENTS

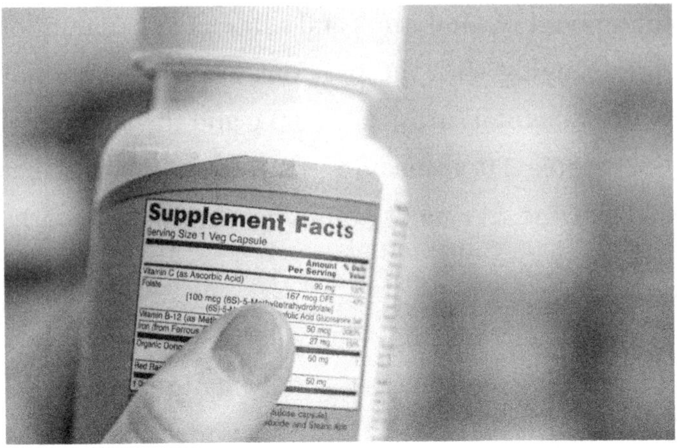

A ketogenic lifestyle cuts out a lot of food and vitamins from your diet, such as the vitamin D in milk and fibers that are found in whole grains. Cutting some of these vitamins and minerals from your diet could lead to what is known as the 'keto flu.' The keto flu usually occurs as the body first enters ketosis and can leave you feeling tired, nauseous, and achy.

Adding supplements to your daily regimen can reduce the chances of getting the keto flu. Someone who is following a ketogenic diet is more likely to have a magnesium deficiency, causing them to experience muscle cramps, high levels of irritability, and trouble sleeping. Using a magnesium supplement, and adding food items that are high in magnesium (like spinach, avocados, and mackerel) can give you a boost in your energy levels, help with your immune system, and reduce your muscle cramps.

Many people believe that even though they are eating cheese and can eat plain Greek yogurt that you are getting enough vitamin D in your diet. However, the restriction of milk and other foods rich in calcium can easily create a deficiency. Adding a daily vitamin D supplement can keep you from feeling fatigued and mentally foggy, while keeping your muscles strong.

Fish and krill oil are packed full of omega-3 fatty acids, like eicosapentaenoic acid (EPA) and docosahexaenoic acid (DHA), that can reduce inflammation in the body and joints, increase your heart health, and help your memory retention. The recommended dosage for the supplement is 1,000 milligrams of DHA and 500 milligrams of EPA per serving. On top of a daily supplement, you can add natural omega-3's by consuming more seafood like salmon, trout, and light tuna.

Vitamins aren't the only innovative supplements that people use for the keto diet. Medium-chain triglycerides (MCTs) have become extremely popular for others who have welcomed the ketogenic diet. They act differently than long-chain triglycerides that are found in fatty foods, as they are absorbed and broken down in your liver and enter your bloodstream as an alternative fuel source for your muscles and brain. Coconut oil is one packed with MCT and is a natural source, rather than a daily supplement vitamin. Some people prefer to use a more concentrated form and use plain MCT oil and add it to their smoothies or their coffee. Supplementing your food with MCT oil is a quick way to increase your daily fat intake and increase the amount of ketones that your body produces. While giving you a kickstart into your ketosis, it also gives you a feeling of fullness throughout the day so you are less likely to grab those last-minute guilty pleasures.

Another way to increase the amount of ketones in your system is to add external ketone supplements. Exogenous ketones give you a boost towards a quicker ketosis, but they have other benefits as well. These benefits include a decreased appetite, an energy boost in your athletic performance, and a faster recovery after workouts.

INTERMITTENT FASTING

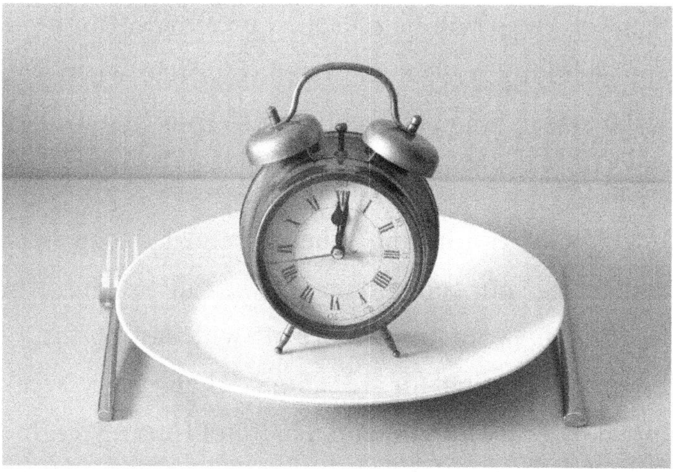

In the section above, you learned that intermittent fasting can be used to get over a plateau. This approach is a scheduled time that you can and cannot eat, and there are quite a few options on fasting times to choose from: 16:8; 12:12; and 14:10. The most popular intermittent fasting approach used is the 16:8, meaning that you fast for 16 hours a day and eat in an allotted 8-hour time period.

You don't have to starve yourself for the entire fasting period, as you can drink water and unsweetened coffee or tea to prevent dehydration and feel full. The number of hours that you sleep through the night counts towards your fasting hours as well, so if you chose the 16:8 schedule, you could eat your first meal at 11 a.m. and stop eating at 7 p.m. The hours that you sleep will help keep your mind off of food, and drinking a glass of water or coffee when you wake up can help you feel full until your first meal of the day.

If you start the fasting schedule and have an issue restricting your food intake for the full 16 hours, try building up your time. Start off with fasting for 12 hours and eating for 12 hours. Then, every week move your fasting time up a half hour until you find a fasting time that you are comfortable with. If fasting for seven days a week is too much for you, try intermittent fasting for five days and have a lower calorie fast (under 500 calories) the other two days.

The reason that intermittent fasting works so well with the keto diet is due to the fact that while you are fasting your body creates ketones. So, if you find yourself having trouble getting into ketosis or are stuck on a plateau, those extra ketones you are gaining can give you the push you need.

AIR FRYERS

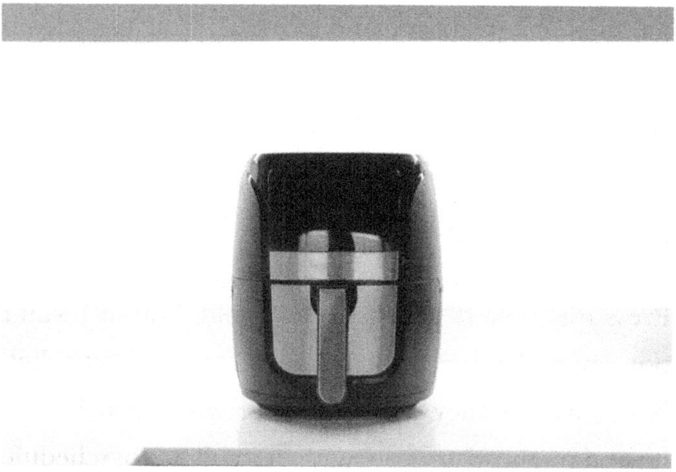

If you don't have an air fryer by now, I highly suggest getting one. Everyone loves crispy food, whether it's zucchini fries or chicken tenders, and you can enjoy these healthy versions sans the calorie-packed oil.

Air fryers cook your food evenly by circulating heat and air without having to submerge your food in oil. The airflow is superheated and gives your food moisture as the fans push the heat around your food. Not only is your food cooked quickly, but you are left with a crunchy outside and a moist center.

Meat isn't the only thing that you can cook in the air fryer, either. You can roast nuts, like almonds, macadamias, walnuts, and peanuts. You can steam your vegetables, like green beans, asparagus, cauliflower, onions, and tomatoes.

INSTANT POTS

Pressure cookers aren't a new trend, but an instant pot can make a world of change for your keto diet. Not only are they a helpful tool when you have a busy day ahead of you with its ability to schedule your cooking time, but it is a godsend during the winter months when you crave some ketogenic hearty soups. An instant pot is also beneficial when it comes to making hard-boiled eggs in 10minutes without waiting for the water to boil.

GUT HEALTH

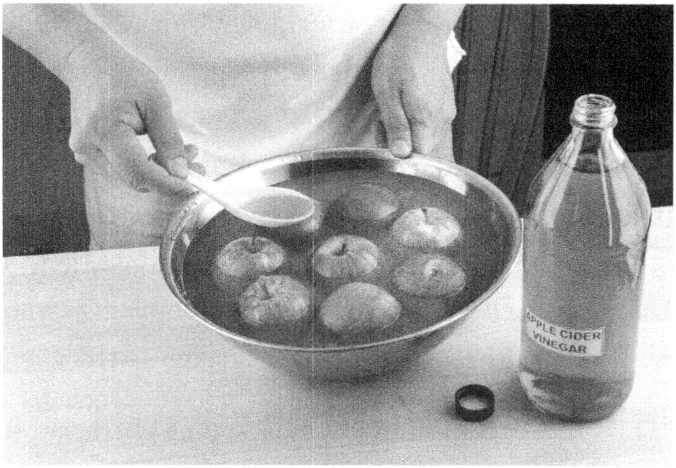

The microbes inside your "gut microbiome" help with a healthy digestion, absorb nutrients, and protect your immune system when it is properly balanced by a healthy diet and exercise. If the microbes aren't properly balanced, you can develop autoimmune issues and get very sick.

So what does the health of your gut have to do with your weight loss? Studies have found that the food that you consume is connected to the health of your stomach and the balance of the microbes. Being overweight and having a deficient metabolism are signs of a damaged gut microbiome, often leading to heart disease and some cancers.

A new study conducted by UC San Francisco in May 2020 has shown the positive impact that the ketogenic diet can have on your gut health. The study found a significant amount of reduction in inflammation due to higher levels of ketones. It also indicated that a ketogenic diet could be a potential treatment for irritable bowel syndrome (IBS) and other autoimmune disorders that affect digestion. A UCSF associate professor and microbiologist who was a part of the study, Peter Turnbaugh stated,

"This is a really fascinating finding because it suggests that the effects of ketogenic diets on the microbiome are not just about the diet itself, but how the diet alters the body's metabolism, which then has downstream effects on the microbiome." (Shreiner et al., 2015).

USING APPS FOR YOUR SUCCESS

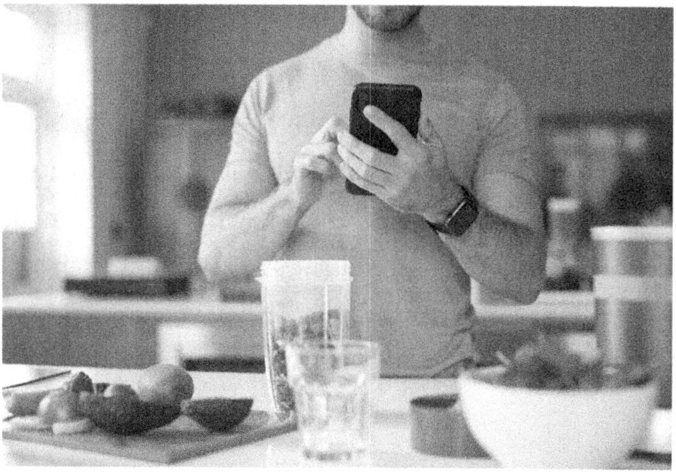

Using smartphone apps can help you in the long run. Whether they are used to count your macros, keep track of your progress, or help you keep time on your fasting hours you can know where you stand throughout the day. Some apps offer delicious recipes containing the macros for each serving, nutritional advice, and a chance to be part of a community of fellow keto dieters.

The features and advantages of each app varies, as well as the experience needed for the user. Most of the apps are free, but many of them have optional premium packages to purchase that unlock more features. Apps like *Carb Manager, Total Keto Diet,* and

Senza are all free to download; can scan an ingredient's barcode for quicker tracking; and provide various keto recipes for meals, desserts, and beverages. Apps like *MyFitnessPal* track your calories and can sync with your fitness watch to track your steps and calories burned. Some apps are strictly focused on recipes only, like *Keto Diet Recipes.* You can be successful in your keto journey by finding which app works best for you and caters to your needs.

3

THE QUICK START GUIDE TO KICKSTART YOU INTO KETOSIS

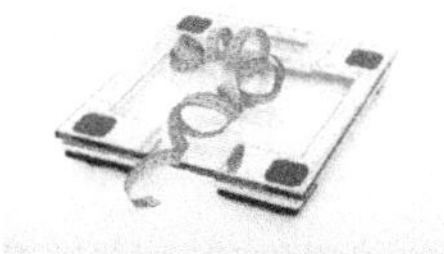

Knowing what you should and shouldn't eat, using apps to count your macros, and supplementing your vitamins is all fine and dandy, but how can you get yourself into a state of ketosis quickly?

7-DAY QUICK RECOVERY TO GET OVER THE KETO FLU

Before you start on your journey into the keto lifestyle, there is one issue that you must be aware of and that is something known as the "keto flu."' When you are cleansing your body of a drug or don't fulfill your body's urges to put that addicting substance in your system, your body goes through withdrawal.

Just like a drug, sugar and carbs can be considered an addiction. Your body relies on carbohydrates and the sugar that it contains to stay balanced. Take that away and your body goes haywire. That is when the keto flu comes into play. The symptoms of the keto flu, sometimes referred to as the carb flu, vary, but the most commonly reported symptoms are:

- nausea
- cramping
- stomach pains
- severe headaches
- constant thirst and dry mouth
- constipation or diarrhea
- brain fogginess
- poor concentration and inability to focus
- sleeping troubles
- muscle fatigue or soreness
- dizzy spells
- fatigue
- irritability
- strong sugar cravings

In most cases, the symptoms only last about a week, and the onset of these symptoms can start as early as two days after starting the keto diet. However, some people are lucky enough to never experience these symptoms at all. You don't have to suffer from these symptoms as there are some things that you can try to combat the severity until the keto flu subsides.

1. *Keep your body hydrated.* Becoming dehydrated and the loss of minerals that goes along with dehydration can make your symptoms more intense, especially headaches and fatigue. Remembering to drink the recommended amount of water for your body can minimize the symptoms of the keto flu. If you aren't sure how much water you are supposed to be drinking during the day, here is how you calculate it: take your current body weight and divide it in half. That is the minimum number of ounces that you should be drinking during the day. Staying hydrated will also promote a feeling of fullness throughout the day and help with food cravings, especially those pesky sugar cravings.
2. *Supplement your electrolytes.* If you are familiar with the minerals lost during hydration, you will know the importance of supplementing them. Supplementing your

diet with minerals like sodium, magnesium, and potassium can minimize your muscle cramps and nausea that are frequently experienced with the keto flu. Some people find it helpful to drink 8 ounces of chicken, bone, or vegetable broth during the recovery process. You could even add a pinch of salt into your glasses of iced water to ensure that you are getting the sodium that you are missing in your diet.

3. *Add more fats to your daily intake.* One of the crucial steps of the keto diet is increasing the consumption of your healthy fats. People often make the mistake of trying to eat low-carb *and* low-fat foods as a way to lose weight quicker, only to find themselves feeling exhausted and nauseous. Adding large amounts of healthy fats, such as avocados, bacon, and egg yolks, to your meal can make the transition into ketosis a much smoother one.
4. *Catch those Z's.* Just like when you are sick from the traditional flu or cold, you will need your rest. Your body needs time to recuperate from the withdrawal of sugar and carbs, and getting an adequate amount of

sleep can help you feel better. Many people find an amount of energy that they have never experienced before when they are in ketosis, but they still have to make sure that they are getting enough sleep to keep that energy flowing. Getting at least seven to eight hours of restful sleep at night will help you lose weight and increase your ability to focus throughout the day, while increasing your productivity level and motivation to be more active.

5. *Try some light exercise.* Nobody feels like exercising when they feel tired and nauseated; however, with the keto flu a light amount of activity, such as yoga or pilates, can minimize muscle soreness and stomach cramps. Light activity can also help improve your mood and irritability level due to the increased endorphins released when you exercise.

Following these five suggestions are easy ways to alleviate the symptoms of the keto flu, but they can also be used to keep the symptoms away. Making sure that you are hydrated and getting enough sodium and fat in your diet from the very beginning can keep the symptoms at bay in hopes that you never experience the keto flu to begin with.

THE JUMPSTART PLAN FOR BEGINNERS

Keto can be tricky in the beginning, and it's understandable how many can become frustrated. In order to jumpstart yourself into ketosis, there are a few things that you need to do:

1. *Slow and steady wins the race.* Everyone who starts the keto diet feels the need to get themselves into ketosis immediately, and that mentality is what makes them feel sick within a couple days. Your body needs time to adjust to cutting back on your sugar and carbs, so start slow for about a week, and then the next week go full keto. Losing weight and being healthy is a lifelong journey, so there is no need to rush and hurt yourself in the process.
2. *Get your macros on track.* Start cutting back on your carbs. While some people begin with their carb intake at 50 g, cutting back to 25 g is the most popular starting point. While keeping within your carb intake, use

the rest of your daily calorie allowance on protein and healthy fats. Your caloric intake and ratios depend on your goals and activity level. To determine the accurate amount you should be consuming on a daily basis, try inputting your information into an online macronutrient calculator.

3. *Balance your blood sugars.* Aside from using a macronutrient calculator to get your macros on track, purchasing a glucose and ketone meter can be a helpful tool in the beginning. The meter can keep track of your fasting blood sugar, post-meal blood sugars, and your increasing ketone levels.

REBOUND FROM THE 2021 PANDEMIC POUNDS

Diet plans of all types have hit a snag thanks to the pandemic and subsequent quarantines. Don't think you are the only one who may have gained a few pounds because it seemed like most people had an issue with gaining weight during such a stressful time. The Centers for Disease Control and Prevention has reported that the amount of weight gain and obesity in adults has significantly increased to over 40% during the pandemic in the United States alone (Hubbard, 2021).

You may have started strong in the beginning of the pandemic, feeling less concerned about temptations due to restaurant closings and a slight pause in friendly outings, but after a while, the boredom caught up with you. The snacks and sugary food that you had successfully avoided before the pandemic became your comfort, and the pounds started to pile back on. Those pandemic pounds don't have to be a constant reminder of your lack of self-control and a terrible year, as you can restart your diet just like you did in the very beginning. Start slowly cutting down on your carbs, tracking your macronutrients, only buying what you are supposed to be eating, and get active so that you can burn off those extra calories. Gaining some pounds back doesn't mean that your journey is over; it's just the start to a new chapter.

KICKSTART PLAN FOR DIETERS 50+

Dieters over the age of 50 may experience a little difficulty getting themselves into ketosis, but by making some small changes, you can make your dreams a reality. Keep in mind that food is metabolized at a different speed as you age, so you will have to compensate for this by moving around the food ratio just a little bit.

As you read in the first chapter of this book, muscle loss and disintegration occur as you age. On the keto diet, you are going to want to make up for this muscle loss by eating more protein. Protein is going to be a key component for dieters over the age of 50because not only will it increase your muscle mass, but it will help give your metabolism a boost.

You will also want to make sure that you are consuming the right amount of healthy fats with every meal. Figuring out how much fat you should include in each meal without going over your daily caloric intake can assist in your weight loss and feeling full throughout the day. In the beginning, it may be necessary for you to eat high amounts of healthy fats so that your body can become adapted to it and learn to rely on the fats as its main energy source.

Getting older tends to come with an extra amount of stress attached. Stress about finances, retirement, your spouse's health, as well as your own, can become overwhelmingly unhealthy to your body and its progress. High levels of stress equal high levels of the hormone cortisol. This hormone is known for hitting the pause button on one's metabolism, while simultaneously increasing their appetite and cravings for processed food and snacks packed with carbohydrates as a way to cope. Finding ways to cope with your stress level that is beneficial to your progress (such as meditation, nature walks, and yoga), can give you that extra push to get you into ketosis and keep you there.

Be sure to keep a watchful eye on how well you are sleeping. Sleep quality tends to take a nose dive as you age thanks to hormone changes within the body. Keeping a consistent sleep schedule can decrease your cortisol level, boost your energy level, and keep you from a frustrating weight loss plateau.

PREPARING FOR YOUR FIRST WEEK OF KETO

Knowing what to eat and what to avoid when you start the keto diet is simple, but what about when you actually have to go into the store to buy and prepare the ingredients for a week's worth of meals? I have spoken with so many people who are seeking advice on how they can plan their meals for the week, what alternative ingredients they can use, and how much of each ingredient they should buy. There are so many resources online, but nobody has the time to look through every article and blog and hope that they find the answer to the questions they have.

REMEMBER THAT YOU CAN USE ALTERNATIVE INGREDIENTS

The first bit of advice that you need to know when trying to figure out when planning your meals is this: If you don't like or are unable to eat certain types of foods, then don't make them just because they are considered keto-friendly meals. You should enjoy what you eat, so don't waste your time, money, and happiness on food that you aren't going to want to eat. For example, coconut flour is a common ingredient in many keto recipes, but some people don't like the taste of coconut so they swap it out for almond flour. If there is a recipe that you are interested in trying but don't like an ingredient, there are other keto-friendly alternative ingredients that you can use.

PLAN AHEAD

Keep in mind that meal planning requires planning ahead in more ways than one. You need to figure out what meals you want to eat, how each meal and snack will fit into your macro ratios, and the quantity of each ingredient that you will need for all of your recipes. Believe it or not, three pounds of boneless, skinless chicken breast can go a long way if it is portioned out correctly.

Figuring out how to portion your meals with correct weights and serving sizes can transform one large dinner into meals for a few days. Consider buying some sturdy tupperware and a food scale so that meal preparation can go easier and faster. All recipes and food labels tell you how many servings are in your meal. So if you are making your meal plan and the recipe that you plan to make includes four servings, you can then weigh them out and freeze them in separate containers. *Voila!* You now have four meals made for the week.

Meals prepared in advance can be a major advantage, especially with those who have a busy schedule. Knowing what is in the meal, how it will fit into your daily ratios, and that it's already prepared cuts down on the chances that you will make a quick trip through the drive-thru window of your local fast-food restaurant.

TRACK A FEW DAYS IN ADVANCE

Some people may find it beneficial to put all of their meals and snacks into their tracker a few days prior, so that they can make sure that they hit their fat, protein, and carb goals every day. Putting your meals in a tracker a few days prior can be helpful because you know the food plan for that day, already have it prepared, and can adjust it accordingly if something arises. For example, if I know in advance what meals I plan to eat the day before, then I will know that I should have 7.0 carbs left by the end of the day. So if I'm feeling a little hungry and could really use a small snack, I will be fully aware of how much wiggle room I have when I figure out what snack I want.

In Chapter 4, learn how to create a weekly, biweekly, or monthly plan and a grocery list. There are also some delicious recipes that you can make in a hurry!

4

NUTRITION

30-DAY MEAL PLANS

Creating a meal plan shouldn't be stressful. If the thought of making one for an entire month is frustrating, try starting small and creating one for the week and see how that goes. Once you get used to making a meal plan for the week, increase it to a two-week meal plan until you feel comfortable with making one for the entire month.

Here is what a sample meal plan for a week could look like:

Sunday

Breakfast

Unsweetened coffee, fried egg, cheddar cheese slice, sausage patty (32 g fat, 17 g protein, 0 net carbs, 369 calories)

Lunch

Keto chicken nuggets (29.5 g fat, 27.2 g protein, 2.4 g net carbs, 391 calories)

Dinner

Chicken bacon ranch casserole (44.3 g fat, 27.1 g protein, 4.5 g net carbs, 534 calories)

Desert/ Snacks

Pumpkin pie fat bombs (12.1 g fat, 0.7 g protein, 1.0 g net carbs, 113 calories)

Monday

Breakfast

Unsweetened coffee, cinnamon roll pancakes (40.9 g fat, 13.1 g protein, 3.9 net carbs, 436 calories)

Lunch

Baked chicken thighs and veggies (38.7 g fat, 26.2 g protein, 6.2 g net carbs, 487 calories)

Dinner

Chipotle steak bowl (45.1 g fat, 30.8 g protein, 3.8 g net carbs, 560 calories)

Tuesday

Breakfast

Unsweetened coffee, low-carb maple almond granola bars

(27.2 g fat, 8.4 g protein, 5 net carbs, 313 calories)

Lunch

Steak fajita in a lettuce bowl (30.3 g fat, 25.4 g protein, 6 net carbs, 404

calories

Dinner

Spicy shrimp omelet (16.7 g fat, 27.3 g protein, 3.5 g net carbs, 286 calories)

Wednesday

Breakfast

Unsweetened coffee, avocado toad in a hole

(20.1 g fat, 9.3 g protein, 2.7 g net carbs, 244 calories)

Lunch

Crockpot taco soup (46.2 g fat, 26.0 g protein, 5.7 g net carbs, 550 calories)

Dinner

Chicken and sausage jambalaya (50.1 g fat, 29.7 g protein, 8.0 g net carbs, 614 calories)

Desert/ Snacks

Keto mini cheesecake

(16.8 g fat, 4.2 g protein, 1.9 g net carb, 174 calories)

Thursday

Breakfast

Unsweetened coffee, lemon poppy seed pancakes

(28.5 g fat, 25 g protein, 7.3 net carbs, 393 calories)

Lunch

Shrimp scampi (22.9 g fat, 12.9 g protein, 4.1 g net carbs, 278 calories)

Dinner

Chili dog casserole (31.5 g fat, 19.2 g protein, 5.4 g net carbs, 387 calories)

Friday

Breakfast

Unsweetened coffee, chicken and zucchini breakfast quiche

(25.9 g fat, 18.4 g protein, 3.1 net carbs, 322 calories)

Lunch

Keto egg salad (44.2 g fat, 14.6 g protein, 1.5 g net carbs, 469 calories)

Dinner

Slow-cooker meatball (33.6 g fat, 26.0 g protein, 4.5 g net carbs, 433 calories)

Saturday

Breakfast

Unsweetened coffee, bacon, egg, and cheese cups

(9.8 g fat, 10.9 g protein, 0.6 net carbs, 137 calories)

Dinner

Steak and eggs (51.3 g fat, 45.1 g protein, 2.2 g net carbs, 668 calories)

Lunch

Keto quarter pounder (44.2 g fat, 24.5 g protein, 2.2 g net carbs, 517 calories)

Desert/ Snacks

Butter coffee (25.1 g fat, 0.2 g protein, 0 net carbs, 219 calories)

CREATING YOUR WEEKLY GROCERY LIST

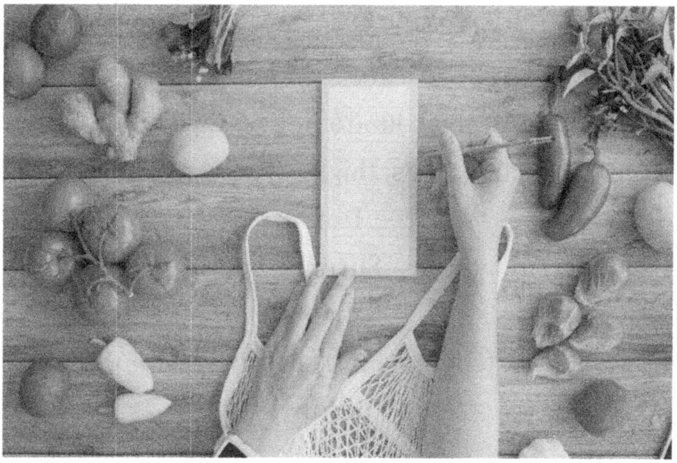

Creating a grocery list becomes an easier task after you make your weekly, biweekly, or monthly meal plan. Knowing what you plan to whip up that week plays a hand in making an effective list so you don't have to keep making a trip to the grocery store. While it isn't unheard of for people or families to go grocery shopping every two weeks, it is highly recommended to plan on going at least once a week to get your fresh berries and vegetables. Fresh produce and unprocessed food have a much shorter shelf life than packaged processed food and meals.

Helpful grocery list guidelines for beginner keto dieters include all the main ingredients for almost every keto meal, besides any special ingredients that you may need for a meal:

Meats/Seafood

Beef (ground/chunks/slabs)

Chicken (breasts, thighs, wings, rotisserie)

Tuna

Shrimp

Salmon

Pork (chops, breakfast sausage, loin)

Bacon

Eggs

Pepperoni

Salami

Tofu

Oils/Fats

avocado oil, extra virgin olive oil, ghee

salted/unsalted butter, nut butters

coconut oil

Dairy

Cheese (shredded, sliced, sticks, blocks)

Cream cheese

Heavy whipping cream

Unsweetened almond milk

Sour cream

Plain greek yogurt

Vegetables

Cauliflower (fresh, frozen, rice)

Broccoli

Kale, lettuce, spinach

Peppers (bell peppers of all colors, jalapeno, banana)

Onions

Eggplant

Cucumber

Zucchini

Spaghetti squash

Garlic (fresh, minced)

Fruits

Strawberries

Blackberries

Raspberries

Blackberries

Avocado

Lemon (fresh, juice)

Snacks

Olives

Nuts (pistachio, almonds, macadamias, peanuts, etc.)

Condiments

Sugar-free ketchup
Mustard
Full-fat ranch
Hot sauce
Broth (chicken, beef, vegetable, bone)
Full-fat blue cheese
Pickle relish
Full-fat mayonnaise

Spices

Salt
Everything but the bagel seasoning
Pepper
Seeds (flax/chia)
Garlic/onion powder
Cumin
Chili powder
Seasoned salt
Coconut/almond flour
Unsweetened cocoa powder
Erythritol/Allulose
Vanilla extract

SIMPLE KETO RECIPES IN UNDER 20 MINUTES

SPINACH, CHEDDAR, AND BACON STUFFED CHICKEN BREAST

2 pounds (32 oz) boneless, skinless chicken breasts, raw
8 oz (1 bar) cream cheese, softened
6 oz (170 g) fresh spinach, ripped into small pieces
1 cup (112 g) shredded cheddar cheese
½ pound (8 oz) of bacon, fried
¼ to ½ cup extra virgin olive oil
¼ teaspoon (0.4 g) garlic powder
¼ teaspoon (0.4 g) onion powder
¼ teaspoon (0.5 g) seasoned salt
¼ teaspoon (0.4 g) chili powder
¼ teaspoon salt
¼ teaspoon pepper

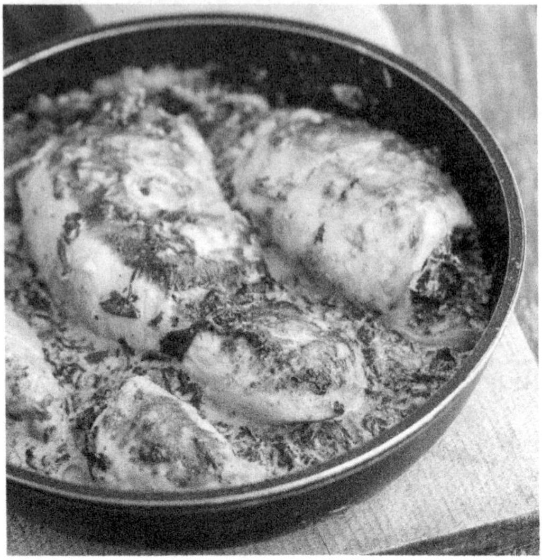

PREHEAT your oven to 400 °F or 204 °C. In a large mixing bowl, mix the bar of cream cheese, the ripped spinach, and shredded cheddar cheese with a hand mixer. Chop up or break your bacon into small pieces and add to the cheesy spinach concoction before mixing with the hand mixer again. Depending on the thickness of the chicken breast, you could cut a pocket into the chicken or fold the chicken breast over and hold the ends together with a toothpick. Spoon the cream cheese mixture into the pocket or on one end of the chicken breast and fold it over. Place the stuffed chicken breasts on some parchment paper placed on a cookie sheet.

In a small bowl, pour about a ¼ cup of extra virgin olive oil into the bottom of the bowl and add the spices into the oil. Mix the spices and oil together and brush the mixture over the chicken breasts. Cook the chicken for 25 minutes or until the center of the chicken breast reaches 165°F or 74°C.

STRAWBERRY JAM

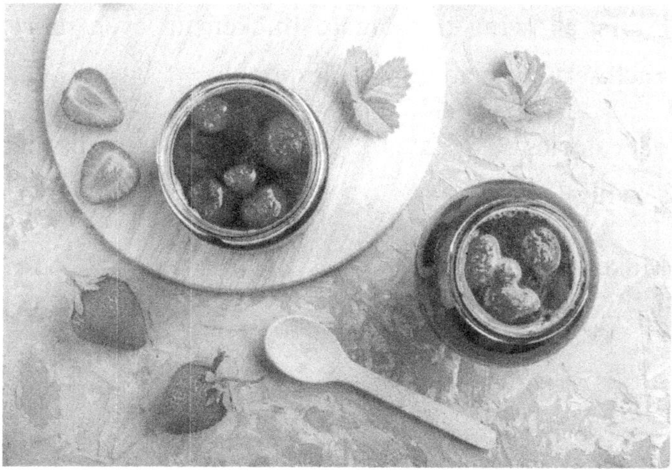

1 pound (16 ounce) bag whole strawberries, frozen
4 tablespoons (50 g) of Pyure erythritol/stevia blend
3 tablespoons (45 g) water
1 tablespoon (15 g) lemon juice

Put all four ingredients into a sauce pan on medium heat. The frozen strawberries will start to release juice and soften. Stir frequently with a fork to avoid burning (strawberry bits tend to get stuck on a whisk). Once the strawberries are completely disintegrated into a sweet liquid, remove the pan from heat to cool. The jam will look thin at first, but will thicken as it cools. Place into a mason jar with a tight lid and put the jar in the freezer for two to three hours, allowing the jam to thicken up even more. Each serving is about 3 tablespoons.

18 calories, 0 g fat, 0 g protein, 3 net carbs per serving

Makes 16 servings

SAUSAGE LOVER'S BREAKFAST CASSEROLE

2 pounds (32 oz) pork breakfast sausage, raw
1 small (70 g) yellow onion, diced
3 cloves (9 g) garlic, minced
2 medium (or 3 small) zucchini, grated
6 large eggs
2 cups (16 oz) coconut milk, canned
salt, to taste
pepper, to taste

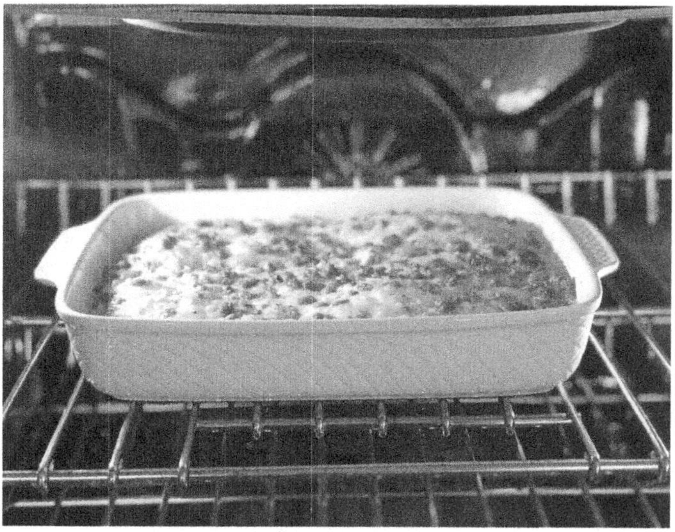

Preheat your oven to 350 °F or 177 °C. Brown the breakfast sausage in a nonstick skillet over medium-high heat. Once the meat is browned, add the onion and garlic and cook until the onions are transparent. Squeeze the grated zucchini between two paper towels to remove any excess moisture and pour into a large mixing bowl. Add your browned sausage and veggie mixture to the grated zucchini and season it with salt and pepper. Stir the ingredients together and spread the mixture evenly into a lightly greased baking dish. In a separate bowl, whisk together the eggs and coconut milk. Pour the eggs and coconut milk mixture over the seasoned sausage and veggie mixture. Bake in the oven for 35–40 minutes until the top is browned and the eggs are cooked completely through.

462 calories, 41.3 g fat, 18.7 g protein, 3.7 net carbs per serving

Makes 10 servings

EVERYTHING BAGELS

1 ¾ cups (196 g) shredded mozzarella cheese
2 oz (58 g) full-fat cream cheese
¾ cup (84 g) almond flour
1 teaspoon (5 g) baking soda
1 egg
pinch of salt
pinch of garlic powder
everything but the bagel seasoning

Preheat your oven to 425°F or 218°C. Measure the mozzarella cheese and cream cheese, placing them in a large microwave-safe bowl. Microwave the cheeses for 45 seconds and stir together. Microwave it for one more minute, stirring together when done until the mozzarella cheese and cream cheese are fully incorporated. Measure the almond flour and fold it into the melted cheese mixture. It's easier to use your hands for this part rather than using a spoon. Fold in the baking soda, salt, and garlic powder while you are folding in the almond flour.

Put your dough to one side of the bowl and crack the egg, placing the egg on the opposite side of the bowl. Use a fork to whisk the egg, blending the egg white and the yolk. Fold the dough into the whisked egg, until it is completely covered and the egg is pulled through the dough. Rinse your hands and make sure they are completely dry so the dough doesn't stick while you try to roll it. Separate the dough into six even portions and start to roll each portion between your hands until the dough looks like a snake and connect the ends together. If the dough keeps sticking to your hands, spray them with a light layer of cooking oil and rub them together.

After all six portions are formed into a bagel shape, sprinkle everything but the bagel seasoning onto a separate plate. Place the bagel dough face-down on the seasoning and press down, so that the seasoning is covering the top of the bagel and place on top of some parchment paper. After the bagels are seasoned, bake in the oven for 10 minutes. Allow them to cool before you eat them, if you can.

217 calories, 17.6 g fat, 11.7 g protein, 2.6 net carbs per bagel

Makes 6 bagels

PHILLY CHEESESTEAK BOWLS

1 pound (16 oz) beef sirloin or sizzle steak, raw and cut into small pieces
1 whole (119 g) green bell pepper, seeded and sliced
1 small (70 g) onion, sliced thin
6 slice (168 g) provolone cheese
5 tablespoons (71 g) unsalted butter, cut in half
½ tablespoon (2.5 g) minced garlic
onion powder, to taste
garlic powder, to taste
salt and pepper, to taste
dried parsley, to taste

Melt 3 tablespoons of unsalted butter in your frying pan. Add your thinly sliced onions to the melted butter and sprinkle with salt and a ½ tablespoon of minced garlic. When the onions are almost transparent, add the sliced green bell pepper to the pan and stir. Salt and pepper the vegetables and cover the pan so they can soften while they cook.

After the vegetables are almost completely cooked, add the rest of the butter and your raw steak to the pan. Stir the meat and the vegetables together, add the rest of the seasoning, and cover to cook, stirring occasionally. Once the meat is completely cooked, lower the heat to simmer and place your provolone cheese on top and sprinkle with dried parsley before covering with the lid. Your meal will be ready to be plated, or bowled, after the cheese melts.

504 calories, 40.2 g fat, 30.2 g protein, 2.8 net carbs per serving

Makes 4 servings

KETO BROCCOLI SALAD

½ pound (8 oz) bacon, fully cooked and chopped (put some bacon grease aside)
1 pound (454 g) fresh broccoli, cut into florets
1 cup (112 g) shredded cheddar cheese
¾ cup (172 g) mayonnaise
1 tablespoon (15 g) apple cider vinegar, or white vinegar
3 tablespoons (42.6 g) erythritol sweetener
¼ cup (68 g) sunflower seeds

Combine mayonnaise, erythritol, and apple cider vinegar into a large mixing bowl. Measure and mix the rest of the ingredients into the dressing. Taste, and add a small amount of bacon grease if it needs more salt or the dressing is too thick.

401 calories, 38.2 g fat, 8.5 g protein, 4.5 net carbs per serving

Makes 5 servings

HOMEMADE MAYONNAISE

250 milliliters (228 gram) extra virgin olive oil
1 tablespoon dijon mustard
1 tablespoon (15 g) lemon juice
1 egg yolk
¼ tsp salt

The best way to make homemade mayonnaise is with a large mason jar and the frothing attachment of an immersion blender. Place the dijon mustard and the egg yolk into the mason jar. Use the frothing attachment and mix until fully combined. Slowly add the olive oil, while mixing consistently so that the emulsion of the ingredients can occur. You may need a second person for this part, one to pour and one to mix. Once the mixture starts to form a stiff consistency, you can start adding the olive oil more quickly. Mix in your lemon juice and salt for a lighter color and better taste.

148 calories, 16.6 g fat, 0.2 g protein, 0.1 net carbs per serving

KETO MEALS TO MAKE IN YOUR AIR FRYER

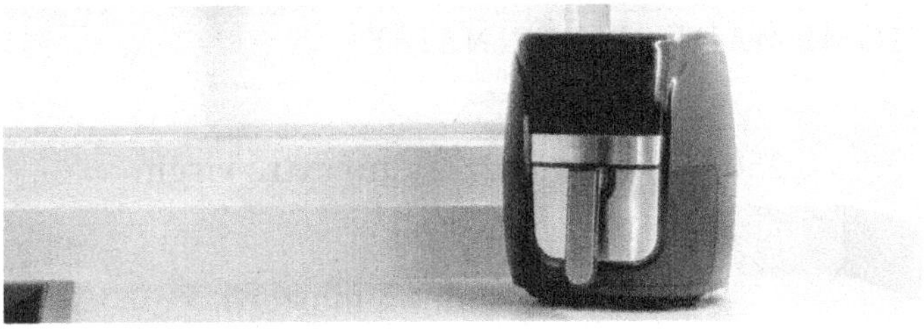

AIR FRYER PARMESAN CHICKEN TENDERS

1 pound (16 oz) chicken breast, cut into strips
¾ cup (85 g) parmesan cheese
¾ cup (84 g) almond flour
1 large egg, whisked
salt and pepper, to taste

Preheat your air fryer temperature to 400 °F or 340°C. In a small mixing bowl, combine the almond flour and the parmesan cheese. Whisk your egg in a separate bowl. Dip the raw chicken strips into the egg and then dredge them into the dry ingredients bowl, ensuring that the chicken strip is covered. After all of the chicken strips are covered, spray them lightly with a mist of cooking spray. Place the chicken strips into the air fryer basket and bake for 17–19 minutes. Chicken strips should be cooked thoroughly and the outside will be brown and crispy upon removal.

376 calories, 25.4 g fat, 32.2 g protein, 2.6 net carbs per serving

Makes 4 servings

ZUCCHINI FRIES

2 medium (392 g) zucchini, fresh
¼ cup (2 oz) heavy whipping cream
1 cup (112 g) almond flour
¾ cup (85 g) parmesan cheese
1 large egg
1 teaspoon (3 g) garlic powder
½ teaspoon (3 g) salt
½ teaspoon (1 g) pepper
½ teaspoon (1 g) paprika

Preheat your air fryer temperature to 400 °F or 340 °C. Slice your zucchini into fry-shaped strips, measuring about 3 inches long and ½ inch wide. In a small mixing bowl, combine the almond flour, parmesan cheese, and spices. Whisk your egg and heavy whipping cream in a separate bowl. Dip the zucchini strips into the egg and cream mixture and then into the dry ingredients bowl, ensuring that each strip is covered. Place the breaded zucchini strips into the air fryer basket and bake for about 10 minutes.

335 calories, 36.4 g fat, 16.9 g protein, 6.4 net carbs per serving

Makes 4 servings

FRIED CHICKEN AND BACON PATTIES

2 whole (238 g) small red bell peppers, cored and seeds removed
10 oz (283 g) boneless, skinless chicken thigh, raw and cut into chunks
3 tablespoons (21 g) coconut flour
¼ cup (28 g) parmesan cheese
4 strips (44 g) bacon, cooked and chopped
1 large egg
salt and pepper, to taste

Preheat your air fryer temperature to 400 °F or 340 °C . Place the red bell pepper into a food processor and pulse until pepper is chopped coarsely. Add the chicken thigh meat and the chopped bacon into the food processor, pulsing until the three ingredients become a smooth mixture. Add the coconut flour, parmesan cheese, egg, and seasoning to the mixture. Pulse all ingredients until they all come together evenly. Once the mixture is well-blended, place it into a large bowl and start to shape out nine identical sized patties. Spray the air fryer basket with a light layer of cooking oil and place two or three patties into the basket, cooking them for about 10 minutes and cooked completely through. Drain the patties on a paper towel and repeat with the rest of the uncooked patties.

363 calories, 24.2 g fat, 27.8 g protein, 4.1 net carbs per serving

Makes 3 servings

AIR FRYER CHICKEN FAJITAS

1 pound (450 g) boneless, skinless chicken breast, cut into strips
1 medium (119 g) yellow bell pepper, cut into strips
1 medium (119 g) green bell pepper, cut into strips
1 medium (119 g) red bell pepper, cut into strips
1 small (70 g) red onion, sliced
1 tablespoon (13.3 g) olive oil
salt, to taste
pepper, to taste
onion power, to taste
garlic powder, to taste
chili powder, to taste
cumin powder, to taste

Preheat your air fryer temperature to 390 °F or 200 °C . While your air fryer heats up, place your chicken strips into a large mixing bowl, drizzle the olive oil, and season the raw chicken to your preference. Toss the chicken and seasoning around in the olive oil until it is well-coated. Add the vegetables, a little more seasoning, and toss again. Put your seasoned mixture into the air fryer and cook for 15 minutes, tossing them around the basket halfway through. Make sure that the chicken is cooked completely before serving. You could eat them with low-carb tortillas or as a salad with some lettuce.

154 calories, 10 g fat, 11 g protein, 3 net carbs per serving

Makes 8 fajitas

KETO MEALS TO MAKE IN YOUR INSTANT POT

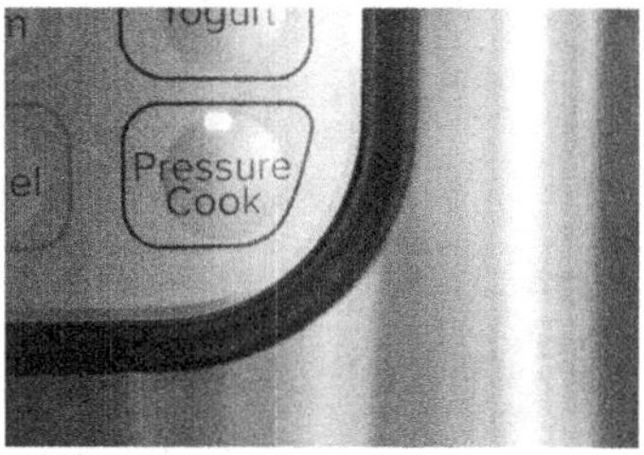

BEEF AND NOODLES

2 to 3 pounds (32 to 48 oz) of beef stew meat
4 cups (32 oz) of beef broth
2 tablespoons beef bouillon powder
½ large (120 g) onion, sliced
sliced mushrooms, optional
¼ cup (2 oz) heavy whipping cream or sour cream
xanthan gum, for thickening preference
salt, to taste
pepper, to taste
onion powder, to taste
garlic powder, to taste

Noodles

2 oz (57 g) cream cheese
4 tablespoons (56.8 g) unsalted butter
4 tablespoons (24 g) of almond flour
3 eggs, whole
pinch of salt

Throw your beef stew meat, broth, onions, sliced mushrooms, and seasoning into your instant pot. Cook for 1 ½ hours on the high-pressure cooking setting. Once the meat is fully cooked, turn the instant pot onto the slow cooker setting for four to five hours. The beef stew meat will become nice and tender, so you don't have to stir it often at risk of the beef chunks falling apart. When the slow cooking time is done, sprinkle a ¼ teaspoon of xanthan gum and stir gently. Replace the lid and check on the thickness in 10 minutes. Add another ¼ teaspoon of xanthan gum and stir, resetting your pressure cooker to cook for 10 minutes on the low setting. Quick release when the 10 minutes are over, and stir the thick broth well. Add ¼ cup of heavy whipping cream or sour cream and stir again.

Twenty minutes before the soup is done, it is time to cook up the noodles! Preheat your oven to 300°F, or 150°C. Add all of your ingredients in a blender, or a Nutribullet, and blend them until the mixture starts to thicken up. Place parchment paper on top of a cookie sheet and pour the mixture onto the parchment paper. Spread out the mix with a spatula so that it is spread evenly. Bake in the oven for 9-10 minutes, and then place it aside to cool down. Once the sheet of your baked mix is cooled, take a pizza cutter and slice your noodles to the preferred size. Place your newly sliced noodles in the crockpot 10 minutes before you eat, so they do not become soggy.

CHICKEN NOODLE SOUP

Two pounds (32 oz) frozen or fresh boneless, skinless chicken breast
4 cups (32 oz) of chicken broth
¼ large (70 g) onion diced or sliced to preference
10 (114 g) baby carrots, or 2 large baby carrots, cut into slices
kosher salt, to taste
pepper, to taste
dried parsley, to taste
onion powder, to taste
garlic power, to taste

Noodles
2 oz (57 g) cream cheese
4 tablespoons (56.8 g) unsalted butter
4 tablespoons (24 g) of almond flour
3 eggs, whole
pinch of salt

Throw the chicken breasts, broth, and seasoning into the instant pot and cook them on high in the pressure cooker setting for 1 ½ to 2 hours. When the pressure cooker is done cooking, carefully release the pressure and add in your vegetables. Set the instant pot into the slow cooker setting for three to four hours.

Twenty minutes before the soup is done, it is time to cook up the noodles! Preheat your oven to 300°F, or 150°C. Add all of your ingredients in a blender, or a Nutribullet, and blend them until the mixture starts to thicken up. Place parchment paper on top of a cookie sheet and pour the mixture onto the parchment paper. Spread out the mix with a spatula so that it is spread evenly. Bake in the oven for 9–10 minutes, and then place it aside to cool down. Once the sheet of your baked mix is cooled, take a pizza cutter and slice your noodles to the preferred size. Place your newly sliced noodles in the crockpot ten minutes before you eat, so they do not become soggy.

KETO CRACK CHICKEN

1 pound (16 oz) boneless, skinless chicken breasts
8 oz (1 bar) cream cheese, softened to room temperature
½ pound (8 oz) bacon, raw and diced
1 cup (8 oz) chicken broth
1 tablespoon (13.3 g) olive oil
1 teaspoon (3.1 g) garlic powder, halved
½ teaspoon (1.5 g) smoked paprika
½ teaspoon (1.5 g) onion powder
½ teaspoon (0.5 g) dill weed
½ teaspoon (0.5 g) dried chives
salt and pepper, to taste

Press the button for the saute setting on your instant pot, and allow it to heat up for a few minutes. Toss your raw, diced bacon in and fry it for two to three minutes until the bacon bits reach preferred crispness. Add the tablespoon of olive oil and give it a few minutes to heat up while you season the chicken breasts with paprika, half the garlic powder, salt, and pepper. Once the olive oil is hot, brown your chicken breasts on both sides. It should take about 2 minutes per side. Press the 'cancel' button to stop sauteing, and in a large mixing bowl combine the room temperature cream cheese, the rest of the garlic powder, onion powder, dried chives, dill weed, salt, and pepper. Mix until ingredients are fully combined and add the mixture to the instant pot. Pour in the cup of chicken broth and pressure cook for 13 minutes on the high setting. Quick release when the time is over and use a fork or hand mixer to shred the chicken breast. Place the instant pot on the "keep warm" setting until the sauce reaches desired thickness. You can enjoy this dish on top of lettuce, low-carb tortillas, or as a vegetable dip.

471 calories, 35 g fat, 32 g protein, 4 net carbs per serving

Makes 4 servings

ITALIAN SAUSAGE KALE SOUP

1 pound (16 oz) mild or hot italian sausage links, removed from casing
1 cup (160 g) white onion, diced
6 cloves (18 g) garlic, minced
12 oz (340 g) cauliflower, frozen
12 oz (340 g) kale, frozen
½ cup (2 oz) heavy whipping cream
½ cup (50 g) shredded parmesan cheese
3 cups (24 oz) water

Press the button for the saute setting on your instant pot, and allow it to heat up for a few minutes. Add the italian sausage and break it up with a wooden spoon while you brown it, as if it were hamburger. Once the sausage starts to brown, toss in your onions and garlic and mix the ingredients together. It's okay if your sausage is cooked all the way through, the instant pot will finish it off for you. When the sausage and chopped vegetables are mixed together, throw your frozen cauliflower and kale in there as well. You don't have to mix in the frozen veggies, as they will mix while cooking.

Add 3 cups of water and start up your pressure cooker for 15 minutes at the normal setting. Let the instant pot release the steam naturally when the time is done, and stir in your ½ cup of heavy whipping cream when it is safe to do so. If you would like your soup to be a little thicker, use your spoon to mash up some of the cauliflower. Pour your hot soup into bowls and top it off with some shredded parmesan cheese before you enjoy.

400 calories, 33 g fat, 16 g protein, 7 net carbs per serving

Makes 6 servings

PLANT-BASED ALTERNATIVE MEALS

AVOCADO POPS

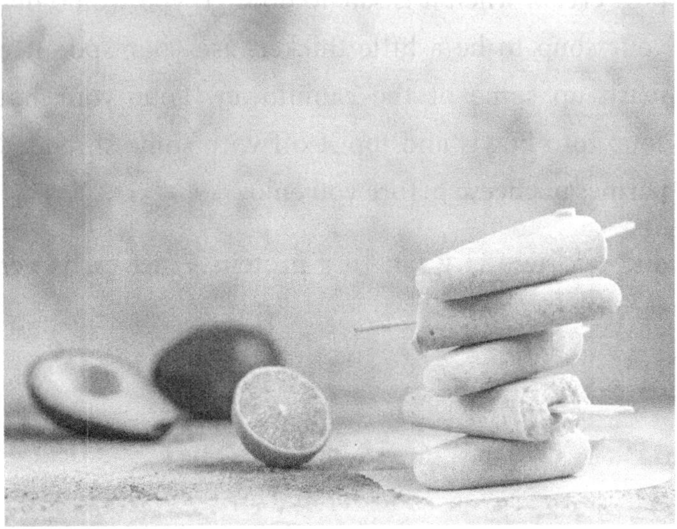

2 medium (300 g) avocados
1 cup (8 oz) unsweetened almond milk
6 tablespoons (85.2 g) of sweetener alternative of your choice
2 tablespoons (30 g) lemon or lime juice

Combine the avocados, almond milk, sweetener, and lemon/lime juice using a blender or food processor until ingredients are blended smoothly. Pour into popsicle molds and place the mold in the freezer. If you would like a little extra sweetness added to your popsicle, melt some sugar-free chocolates with a small amount of butter or cacao butter and dip your frozen treat into the chocolate. You could eat it like that or throw the chocolate dipped delights into the freezer again.

33 calories, 3 g fat, 1 gram protein, 1 net carb per popsicle

Makes 6 popsicles

GUACAMOLE

4 whole (600 g) avocados, ripe and pitted
½ (35 g) of a small onion, finely chopped
1 cup (946 g) fresh cilantro, finely chopped
1 small lemon, zest and juice
1 small lime, zest and juice
2 tomatoes, chopped and seeds removed
½ teaspoon (1.4 g) minced garlic
½ teaspoon (2.5 g) sea salt
¼ teaspoon pepper
cumin and chili pepper, to taste, optional

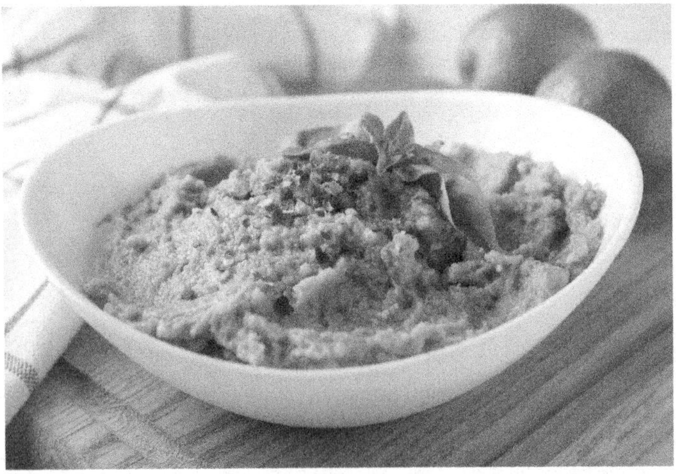

Cut all four of your avocados in half, and remove the pits. Scoop the ripe flesh from the skins and place it into a large mixing bowl. Add the zest and the juice from the lemon and the lime, sea salt, and black pepper to the mixing bowl. Mash the ingredients together with a fork, or you can mix it all together with a food processor. Once the avocado flesh and the flavorings are mixed together, add the chopped ingredients. Stir the ingredients together until they are distributed evenly throughout the bowl and enjoy.

If you keep the pits of the avocados, you can refrigerate them in the bowl with the guacamole so it will stay fresher longer.

113 calories, 10 g fat, 2 g protein, 2 net carbs

Makes 12 servings

ZUCCHINI NOODLES WITH AVOCADO SAUCE

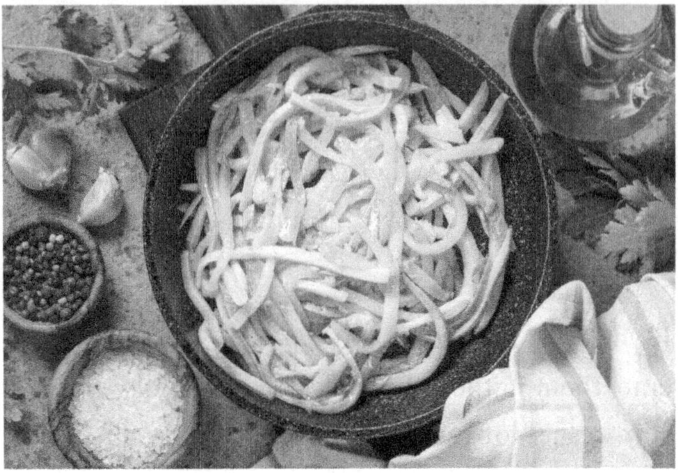

3 large (or 4 medium) zucchinis, spiralized

1 whole (150 g) avocado, ripe and pitted

⅓ cup (315 g) fresh cilantro, coarsely chopped

3 cloves (9 g) of fresh garlic, crushed

1 tablespoon (15 g) lemon juice

¼ cup (2 oz) extra virgin olive oil

½ teaspoon (3 g) salt

¼ teaspoon pepper

water, if needed

cilantro, to serve

parmesan cheese, to serve

After spiralizing the zucchini, place aside on a paper towel so the zoodles can dry. Combine the avocado flesh, lemon juice, half of the olive oil, cilantro, salt, and pepper in a food processor and blend into a smooth puree. If the puree's consistency is too thick, try adding a little water until it meets the consistency of a salad dressing.

Pour the rest of your remaining olive oil into a nonstick frying pan and place above high heat. When the oil is warmed up, throw in your zucchini noodles to saute for about three minutes. Once your zoodles are tender, remove the pan from the heat and pour your avocado sauce over them. Stir the sauce into the noodles gently and top with parmesan cheese and a pinch of fresh cilantro before serving.

245 calories, 22 g fat, 4 g protein, 5 net carbs

Makes 4 servings

RATATOUILLE

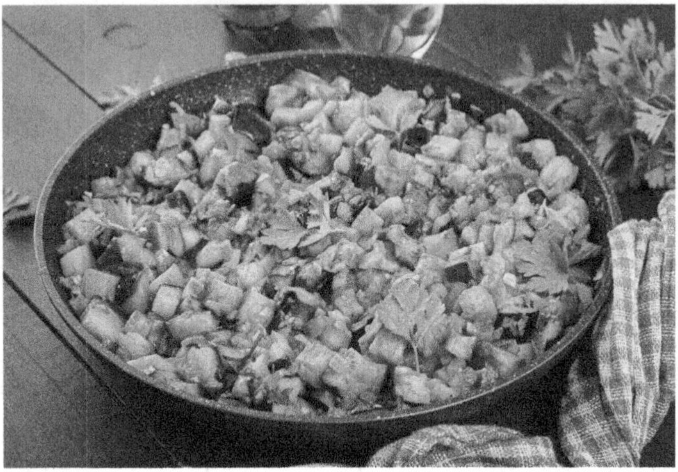

½ of a medium (70 g) red onion, chopped
1 large (660 g) eggplant, chopped
1 large (323 g) zucchini, chopped
1 cup (8 oz) of canned tomato sauce
½ cup (4 oz) water
1 tablespoon (13.3 g) extra virgin olive oil
1 teaspoon (2.8 g) minced garlic
salt, to taste
pepper, to taste

Simmer the red onion in extra virgin olive oil and garlic for about five minutes until it softens. Then, add the eggplant, zucchini, canned tomato sauce, water, and Italian seasoning. Stir the ingredients together and cook over medium heat for 15–20 minutes. Sample the food, add salt and pepper if it's needed. Garnish with some fresh cilantro and enjoy!

66 calories, 3 g fat, 2 g protein, 6 net carbs

Makes 4 servings

5

HEALTH AND FITNESS WITH KETO

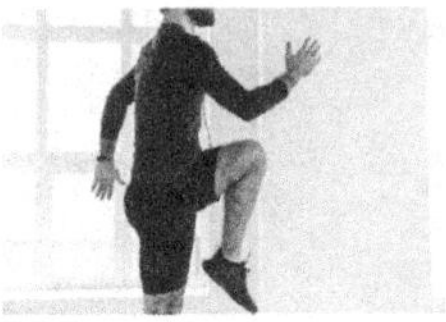

Becoming physically fit while you are on the keto diet has its own set of benefits. Working out while you are on a ketogenic diet increases your muscle mass, slows down the aging process, and minimizes age-related bone loss. A high-fat, low-carb diet, coupled with activities like jogging, bicycling, and aerobic exercise, have been found to be beneficial in burning body fat. Many endurance athletes prefer to add ketone supplements while they are in ketosis as an added boost in their energy level and to decrease their recovery time between workouts.

THE BEST KETO EXERCISES AND WORKOUTS

HIGH-INTENSITY INTERVAL TRAINING (HIIT)

HIIT exercises increase your endurance and performance while getting you into a "fat-burning zone." This workout style gives you the benefit of raising your heart rate, increasing your blood flow, and giving your weight loss a push in the right direction.

HIIT exercises include:

- Push-ups
- Lunges
- Sit-ups
- Burpees
- Sprints
- Jumping rope

Building Up Your Core

The keto diet helps make building our core a little easier. Strengthening your stomach muscles can't be done without a proper diet and exercise plan. However, to build up those hidden abdominal muscles you need to avoid the unhealthiest fat of all — unsaturated fats. Rather than helping you gain muscle, unsaturated fat makes you gain weight. Abdominal exercises also help you burn fat around your waist and build up your endurance for other activities.

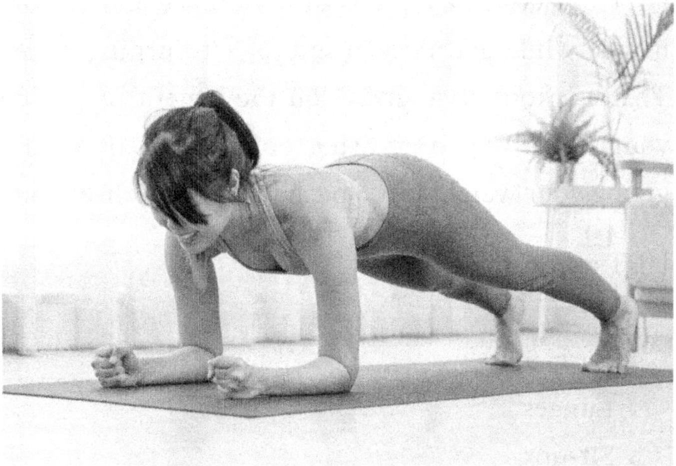

Exercises that can help you build up your core include:

- Planks
- Mountain climbers
- Lying leg raises
- Russian twists
- V-sit-ups

KETTLEBELL AND BARBELL TRAINING

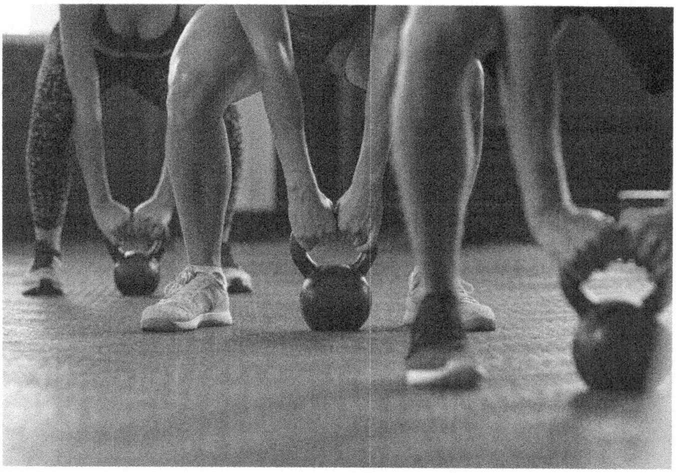

Kettlebell and barbell workouts have awesome benefits when it comes to your overall health and physical well-being. Just to name a few of these amazing benefits: improving your posture, flexibility, and heart health; building muscle, functional strength, cardio fitness endurance; boosting your balance; and goes easy on your back and spine.

Kettlebell and barbell training exercises include:

- Barbell
- Squats

- Deadlifts
- Bench presses
- Standing bicep curls
- Overhead shoulder presses
- Closed grip bench presses
- Kettlebell
- Swings between the legs and hand-to-hand
- Squats
- Suitcase lunges
- Deadlifts
- Sumo deadlifts with high pulls
- Push presses
- Figure 8's

BENEFITS YOU CAN GAIN FROM WALKING, YOGA, AND OTHER LOW-IMPACT EXERCISES

Low-intensity workouts can do wonders for your weight-loss journey. These exercises build up your energy level while the body burns calories and allows it to use fat as its fuel source. They also give your endurance a boost so that your body as your heart rate increases and creates more ketones thanks to your stored body fat.

Benefits of walking daily include:

- Lowers your risk of a stroke and/or heart attack and disease
- Strengthens your joints and bones
- Reduces inflammation in your joints
- Reduces hypertension and cholesterol levels
- Reduces body fat
- Aiding management of diabetes
- Increases your lung capacity
- Great for socialization

Benefits of yoga include:

- Improves your flexibility, balance, and strength
- Manages and minimizes your stress level
- Improves your energy level and your mood
- Better sleep quality and makes you feel more relaxed
- Improves your breathing and heart health
- Strengthens and tones all of your muscles
- Gives your metabolism a boost
- Improves mental health
- Helps maintaining your blood sugar
- Improves your posture
- Aids in weight loss

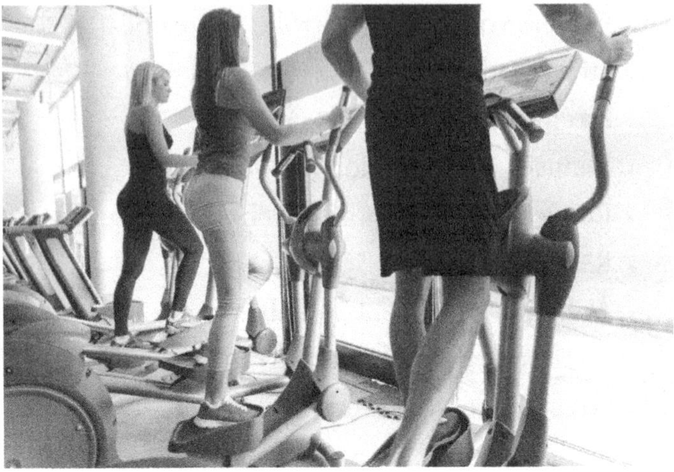

Benefits of elliptical training include:

- Boosts your stamina
- Strengthens your muscles, lungs, and heart
- Burns calories and body fat
- Less stress on your achy joints and past injuries
- Works out all parts of your body
- Targets specific leg muscles (glutes, hamstrings, calves, and quads)
- Improves your balance and recovery speed from injuries

Benefits of swimming and water aerobics include:

- Less stress on joints, arthritis, and previous injuries
- Less strain on your heart muscle
- A greater range of motion thanks to the water
- Builds strength by having to work against the water
- Allows you to stay cool so you can work out longer

Benefits of stationary bicycling include:

- Boosts your heart rate and cardio fitness
- Burns as much as 300 calories in only 30 minutes
- Builds and tones your leg muscles
- Strengthens muscles in your lower body
- Burns body fat
- Eases stress and reduces joint inflammation
- Strengthens your lungs and utilizes more oxygen
- Boosts energy and decreases daily fatigue

6

STAYING ON TRACK AND KEEPING YOURSELF ACCOUNTABLE

FIND YOURSELF AN ACCOUNTABILITY BUDDY!

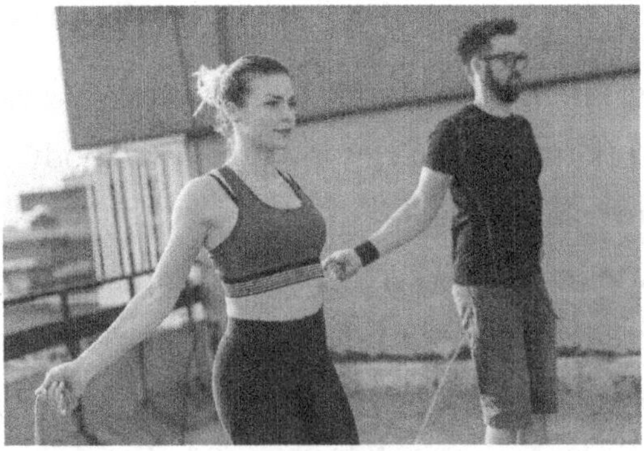

A healthy weight-loss accountability buddy relationship can be difficult to find. There are some awesome benefits to having an accountability buddy, like providing support, motivation, and encouragement when you feel like you can't go any further in your journey. However, the difficult part of the relationship comes into play when selecting the right buddy.

When finding a good accountability partner, you will want to make sure that this person is reliable in other aspects of life. Do they show up on time and when they are supposed to? Can you count on them to show up, or are they flakey? Do they have a successful track record with losing weight or helping others lose weight? How are this person's weight-loss goals similar or different to yours? Ensuring that you pick the right person as an accountability partner can go a long way when it comes to being successful in weight loss and having a great support system.

TRACKING FOR SUCCESS

Tracking is a great way to hold yourself accountable for your weight loss and what you ate that day. Keeping track of how much weight you have lost can become an excellent source of motivation. Watching that number rise inspires you to keep going as you get closer to your goal weight.

When it comes to tracking your food, everyone's experience and choices on what to track vary. Some dieters prefer to be strict on their diet and track every item and drink that they put in their mouth, while others don't calculate certain foods like low-carb vegetables. This thought process was explained to me by a close friend when I asked why they didn't track their veggies, they stated, "Vegetables didn't make me fat, so why would I track them?" I laughed when I first heard this statement, but afterwards it started to make a lot of sense. In other words, how strict you are with your tracking doesn't necessarily mean that you will be more successful. However, it will help you hold yourself more accountable, keep track of your macros and calories, and keep yourself motivated as you watch the amount of weight that you have lost increase.

FOOD, MOOD, AND GUT HEALTH

Not only should you be tracking your food to see how you are progressing, you should also track your mood and your gut health. The keto diet isn't all about dropping numbers on the scale and dropping pant sizes; it's about feeling better, happier, and healthier. Are you feeling more energized and fuller throughout the day, or are you feeling grumpy and hungry between meals? Do you struggle with bouts of constipation and feeling bloated?

There are plenty of mood-tracking apps that you can download on your phone if you would like to track your daily patterns. You could see if your moods are shifting at a certain part of the day and adjust your meals or snacks accordingly. If you are feeling constipated or bloated on a regular basis, you may need to increase your water intake and consume foods that have a higher fiber content.

SETTING REALISTIC GOALS

It is of utmost importance to set a realistic goal for yourself when you are dieting. Not only will it seem more attainable as you get closer, but a realistic goal will keep you from getting discouraged if you have an off-day or a bad week. If you set a goal that you want to lose 80 pounds in the next month, how would you feel if you don't accomplish that goal at the end of the month? If that goal was considered possible to do, would you be able to do that in a healthy way?

The easiest way to set a realistic goal is to choose a reasonable deadline for losing a certain amount of weight. If we are using the example of wanting to lose 80 pounds and you are starting at the beginning of the year, a realistic and attainable deadline for your goal would be the beginning of the next year or around the holidays. Once you choose a date, set small goals along the way, such as losing two to three pounds a week or 10 pounds a month.

To keep you motivated while you are moving towards your goal, set up small rewards that don't revolve around food when you meet your weekly or monthly goal. Go to the movies with your friends, or go bowling with your kids. Give yourself something to look forward to, especially when you reach your goal weight at the end of your deadline. Schedule a vacation or an activity that you were too afraid to do before you lost weight. Remember to celebrate the small victories along with the big ones—you earned it.

NAVIGATING KETO WITH YOUR FAMILY

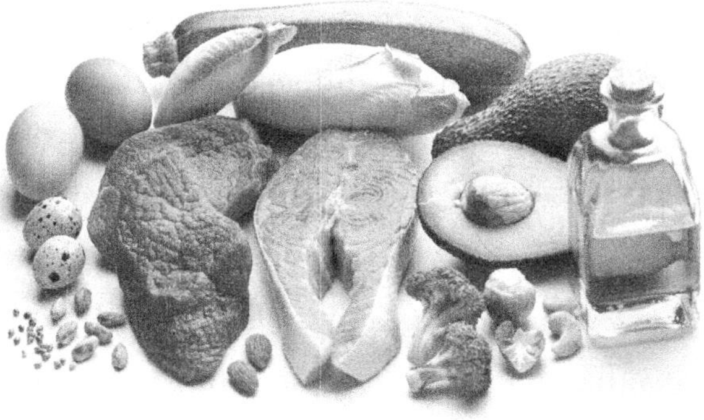

Going on a diet when you are the only person in your house is easy compared to when you have children to feed as well. Who wants to cook two meals at the same time? Would you really want to watch your children eat your favorite meal, or hear the sounds of them spitting out your bland food when they want something delicious?

That's the amazing thing about keto! It takes all of the ingredients that you and your family love and puts them in a fulfilling, satisfying diet. Cheesy scrambled eggs and bacon for breakfast? Yes, please! Almonds, pepperoni, and sliced up cheese sticks with a strawberry smoothie for a snack? What kid wouldn't love that?

Providing children with an education on healthy food and staying active will give them the information that they will need when they grow up and are on their own. Most of the meals are easy to make, so you could easily make dinnertime a family affair with cooking lessons for younger children. Getting your entire family involved makes the keto diet easier to stick with. However, don't forget that there are some vitamins and minerals that children need to grow, like the vitamin D that they get from milk, so they will need to be supplemented appropriately.

AVOIDING DIET TRAPS

The dieting world is filled with so many traps, ranging from hidden sugars and carbs to food marketed directly for your diet. People assume that just because the front of the package says sugar-free that the food is safe on the keto diet. However, there are other names for these artificial sweeteners that can stall your progress. The list of hidden artificial sweeteners to look for on food labels include:

- Aspartame
- Xylitol
- Sorbitol
- Maltitol
- Dextrose
- Splenda

Enjoying foods that include these hidden sugars, sometimes referred to as sugar alcohols, can be done every once in a while. However, making them a part of your everyday routine can create a weight-loss plateau or keep you from getting into ketosis. Many of the foods that are marketed towards keto dieters are packed with hidden sugars, and they aren't always as keto friendly as the label promises. Knowing what is in your food is just as important as how much you are eating.

WHERE THE 'SUGAR' DEMON HIDES

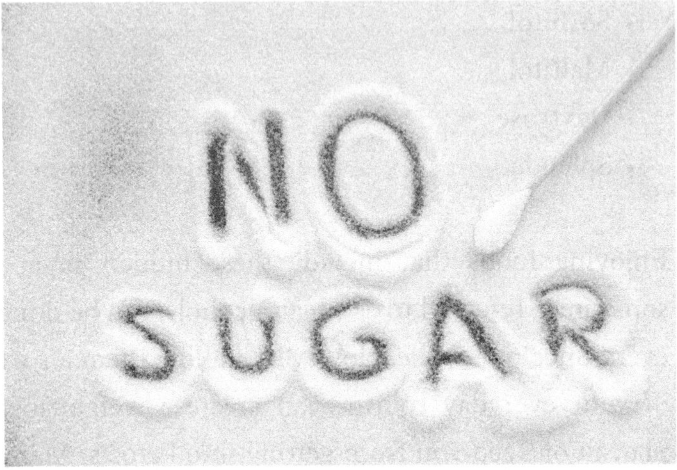

Now that you know the multiple names of sugars to avoid, you should know where these hidden sugars are often found:

- Sugar-free candy
- Non-dairy milks
- Sugar-free soda
- Light salad dressings
- Sauces
- Fruits
- Smoothies

These foods are marketed to soothe those sugar cravings that one can experience when they give up carbs, but consuming too much of them only makes abstaining harder. You aren't technically giving up sugar or glucose. It is just being replaced by other forms of sugar.

If you are in need of an all-natural sweetener, try one that is made of an erythritol/stevia blend or allulose. Brands like Swerve or Pyure are made out of the erythritol/stevia blend and are free of the hidden sugars found in other artificial sweeteners. This allows you to make your favorite snacks without sacrificing flavor or your daily carb limit.

HOW TO DEAL WITH SUGAR CRAVINGS

If you are familiar with how the body works, then you are aware that our body relies heavily on sugar and the sugars that our body extracts from consuming carbohydrates. So when you cut down the amount of sugar and carbs that you are consuming, your body feels like it is going haywire, especially for the first few weeks while you become accustomed to relying on fat rather than carbs. However, there are times after the initial carb withdrawal that you may find yourself craving sugar. The reasons your sweet tooth may be working overtime include:

- Overexerting yourself during workouts
- Not eating enough fat or protein
- Inadequate sleep
- Dehydrated
- Depressed and overstressed

Simple fixes, like readjusting your macros, drinking more water packed with electrolytes, and getting between seven to nine hours of sleep, can be the cure to those insatiable sweet cravings. Remember the keto diet does have some delicious recipes that can minimize your sugar cravings and put some more fat and proteins into your daily consumption; these snacks are most commonly known as fat bombs.

7

BOUNCE BACK STRONGER

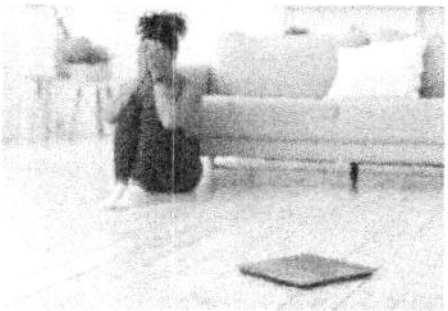

WHAT IS A PLATEAU?

As you lose weight, your metabolism starts to slow down and the number of calories that you burn throughout the day starts to decline, which is why you hit a plateau. There is also the possibility that the reason for your plateau is because you need to reevaluate, and possibly recalculate, your macronutrient ratios.

You may not be tracking your macros closely enough, or the ratios you are currently using aren't working in your favor. The ratio that your body needs could require that you cut your carb intake lower than 10%.

Or you may need to cut back on your protein intake and increase your fat content intake. Carbohydrates and protein are converted into glucose, and having too much glucose in your system can kick you out of ketosis. The ratios are not a set requirement, but they are the basis of where to start for the diet. Since everyone is different, your ratio of fats, proteins, and carbs may need to be tweaked to get you back into ketosis.

Plateaus can also happen when you are eating too many calories during the day. High-fat foods also mean high-calorie food, making it harder to create a calorie deficit. If you aren't burning as many calories as you consume throughout the day, a calorie deficit is impossible to create and kicks you out of ketosis. Other factors that could boot you from being in ketosis are not getting enough sleep and high stress levels.

HOW TO RESET KETOSIS WHEN YOU HIT A PLATEAU

Weight loss isn't always a steady ride, as there are many bumps and hills along the way. Eventually, you will hit a plateau. If you have lost any weight on other diets, know that keto isn't any different. There will be small spans of time that you won't lose any weight. This is about the time that people normally get frustrated and want to give up on their diet, but don't throw in the towel just yet. You can reset your ketosis and get over that plateau.

There is one possible reason that you could be experiencing a plateau, and that is a phenomenon called the "whoosh effect." There are multiple studies that are trying to figure out what causes the effect, because the reasons how and why it happens are still unknown. However, it is theorized that due to the loss in weight and a major change in your diet, your body is attempting to keep itself in balance. So in order for the body to stay in balance, your fat cells will fill with triglycerides to be used for energy because your body thinks it is in starvation mode.

When you consistently keep up with your calorie deficit, your body realizes that it's not in starvation mode and the fat cells will release the triglycerides. After a week or so of being stuck on the same number, you will step on the scale and be surprised to see that you lost up to five pounds seemingly overnight.

So how do you break the plateau? Look for hidden sugars and carbs in your food. Artificial sweeteners have different names that you may think are healthier than regular sugar, but they can have an adverse effect on your weight loss. You could also try adding intermittent fasting, which could speed up your transition back into ketosis. Try adding supplements and exogenous ketones to your daily regimen.

Remember that stress levels can cause a plateau, and a plateau can create stress and frustration. However, just because you aren't seeing a change in the numbers on the scale doesn't mean that you aren't losing inches, weight, or body fat. You may notice that your clothes are getting looser even though the number is still the same. Your mood could be better, energy level is higher, and your blood sugar and cholesterol numbers are in the normal range. All of these things are non-scale victories and show that the diet is working, and you may just need to be patient.

AVOIDING KETO BURNOUT…CHANGE IT UP!

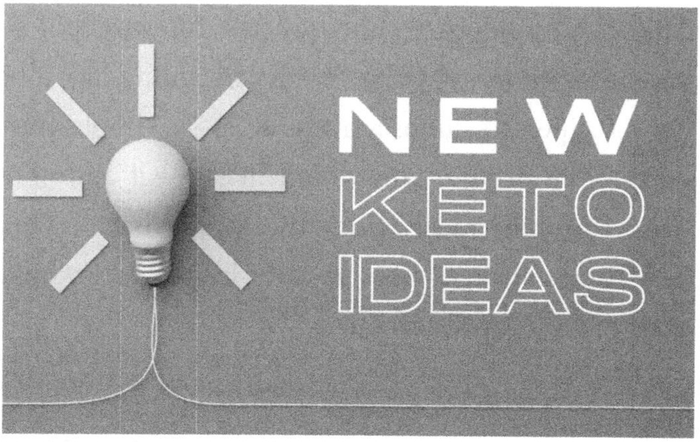

Having a predictable routine is nice, but it can easily become mundane and leave you feeling complacent in your dieting journey. Wondering how long you need to eat this way or how you can keep yourself from losing interest in the keto lifestyle can destroy the strongest-willed dieter's motivation to stay on track. So what can you do to avoid a keto burnout? You change up what you are doing!

MAKE IT MORE INTERESTING AND TRY NEW THINGS

Thanks to modern technology, the Internet, phone apps, and Pinterest, there is a never-ending digest of keto recipes to choose from. It is so simple. Just choose the protein you would like to eat and plug "[protein] keto meals" into the search bar. Trying new things always spices up your life, so why would your diet be any different?

ADD SOME NEW SNACKS TO THE MENU

Everyone loves a good snack, but sometimes hard-boiled eggs and celery sticks with ranch just won't cut it. Adding delicious snacks that will not only keep you full, but will keep you in ketosis is a nice adjustment to keep the burnout away.

Try these snacks to keep your keto diet going and burnout at bay:

- 85% (or higher) cacao concentrate dark chocolate
- Olives canned in olive oil
- Beef jerky (preservative and sweetener-free)
- Pork rinds (original flavor)

For an extra delicious treat, try adding a serving of pork rinds to a 1 ½ tablespoons of melted butter and sprinkled with erythritol sweetener and cinnamon or ranch flavoring and shake it up!

- Vegetables dipped in full-fat dressing or nut butters
- Avocado seasoned with salt and lemon juice

REVAMP AND REFRESH THOSE TIRED RECIPES

Sometimes you may like certain recipes and don't want to throw them out, so maybe there are ways that you could give them a whole new life with a replacement ingredient.

For a grain replacement, try:

- A cheese or lettuce wrap instead of a low-carb tortilla
- Using almond flour instead of coconut flour, and vice versa
- Making keto egg noodles instead of zoodles (spiralized zucchini noodles)

For a refreshing sweetener, try:

- Lemon juice as a salad dressing
- A little pumpkin spice and nutmeg with your keto french toast
- Adding some cinnamon to your bulletproof coffee

MEAT OVERLOAD? TRY VEGAN ALTERNATIVES

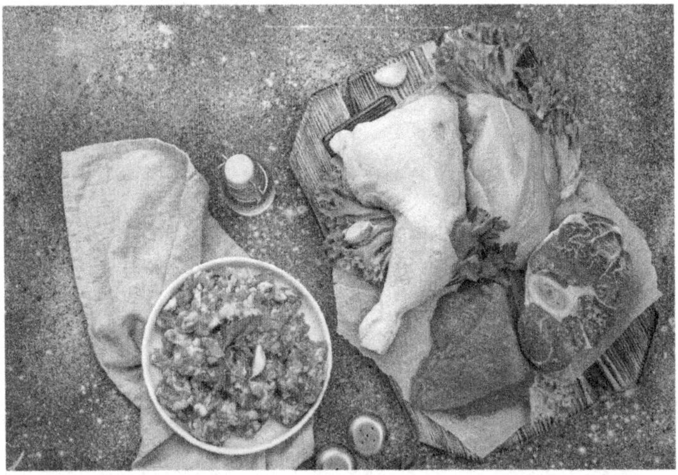

Maybe it's not that you are tired or burnt out on keto, but you are tired of eating the same meaty meals repeatedly. There is no shame in that. However, you could always try doing a vegan keto plan for a while. A vegan keto plan may seem strange, considering the fact that the diet includes the consumption of a large range of proteins throughout the day. However, there are other ways to get in those daily ratios, even with vegan alternatives. Of course, a vegan plan comes with its own set of issues and challenges considering that most of the protein that you ingest comes from eggs, seafood, and cheeses.

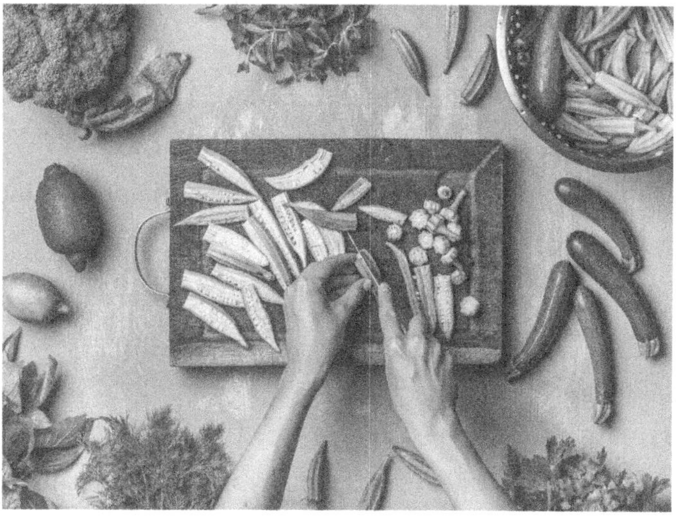

A plant-based ketogenic diet relies on the focus of the non-starchy vegetables that you have learned about in other chapters, like kale, avocados, mushrooms, and olives. You could also get your protein from other sources, such as nuts, seeds, unsweetened almond milk, and coconuts. You could even eat soy-based proteins, like tofu, on occasion. I say "on occasion" because tofu is a processed food and the purpose of a ketogenic diet is to focus on whole foods, but it is okay to enjoy tofu every once and a while.

The vegan, or plant-based, ketogenic plan should be cleared with a doctor due to some complications that may occur. People that struggle with kidney damage, diabetes types I and II, and women who are pregnant or breastfeeding may be at more risk for health problems. Although, women that have PCOS could see some improvement in their symptoms due to the anti-inflammatory benefits of the diet.

GO FISH! RED MEAT ALTERNATIVES

Then again, who said you need to go completely vegan? You could change up your protein source from red meat to seafood. Seafood alternatives can give you a nice boost of the omega-3's that are often forgotten about while people are concentrating on getting their fats and proteins in. Adding more fish alternatives to your menu holds other benefits as well. Seafood is leaner than red meat, high in protein, low in carbohydrates, and contains large amounts of omega-6 and omega-3 fatty acids.

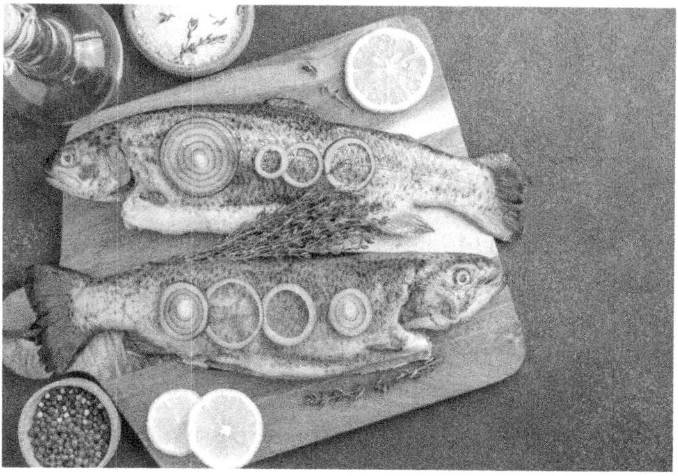

SALMON AND MACKEREL

Salmon isn't just rich in flavor, it's rich in omega-3 fatty acid with over 4,000 mg contained in only half of a fillet. Mackerel contains the same amount of omega-3's but is much milder in flavor than salmon and pairs perfectly with citrus marinades. These hearty filets pack more of a punch vitamin-wise besides the fatty acids. They are also full of vitamin B, vitamin D, and selenium.

GARLIC BUTTER SALMON AND ASPARAGUS

1.5 pounds (24 oz) fresh salmon, cut into 4 fillets

1 pound (453 g) asparagus, ends trimmed

½ cup (8 tablespoons) butter, melted

3 cloves (9 g) garlic, minced

1 tablespoon parsley, minced

1 teaspoon (3.1 g) garlic powder

1 teaspoon (6 g) salt

½ teaspoon pepper

4 slices lemon, thickness cut to preference

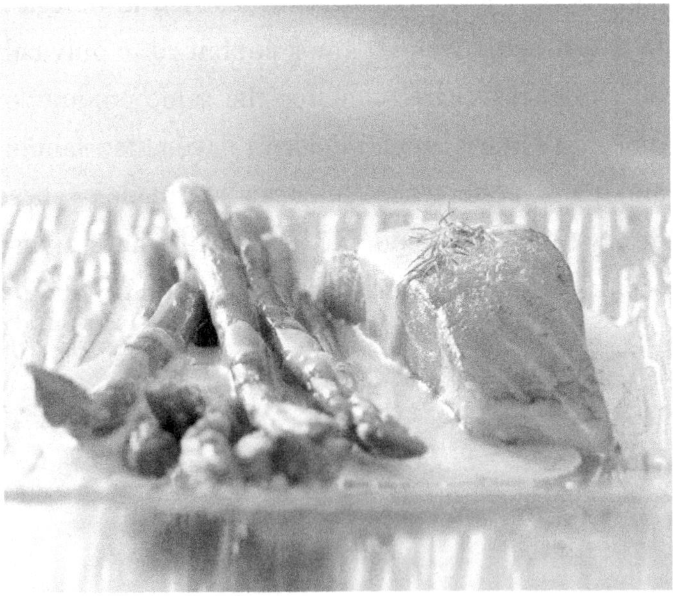

Preheat the oven to 450 °F or 232 °C. Place the salmon fillets into a lightly greased baking sheet, leaving some space between each fillet. Arrange the asparagus around the edges of the baking sheet. In a small mixing bowl, whisk the melted butter, garlic, parsley, and seasonings together. Drizzle the buttery mix over the salmon fillets and asparagus. Place a lemon slice on top of each fillet and bake in the oven for 13 to 15 minutes. The salmon fillet is done when it is tender and opaque in the middle. Serve immediately and enjoy your meal!

587 calories, 44 g fat, 41 g protein, 4 net carbs per serving

Makes 4 servings

EASY MACKEREL PATTIES

14.1 oz (400 g) canned mackerel, drained
½ cup + 1 tablespoon (60 g) almond flour, or
3 tablespoons (24 g) coconut flour
1 tablespoon paleo mayonnaise (or use
homemade mayonnaise recipe from
Chapter 4)
1 large egg, beaten
1 tablespoon (14.9 g) yellow or dijon mustard
1 tablespoon (15 ml) extra virgin olive oil
or ghee
½ teaspoon parsley
½ teaspoon (1.5 g) garlic powder
1 teaspoon (3.1 g) onion powder
sea salt and pepper, to taste

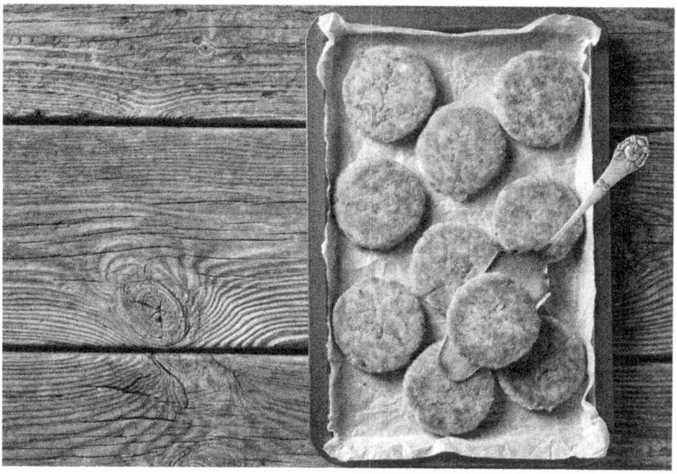

Remove the mackerel from the can and place into a large mixing bowl. Break it up and mash it with a fork. Add the rest of the ingredients, except for the olive oil or ghee and a ¼ cup (25 g) of the almond flour. However, if you decide to use coconut flour, add the entire amount. Mix until all ingredients are distributed throughout. Using a ¼ cup measuring cup, scoop out 9 patties and shape them with your hands. Flatten the patties and coat the outside of each one with the remaining almond flour.

In a large frying pan, pour the extra virgin olive oil or ghee and heat it up over medium heat. Cook 3 patties at a time for about three to four minutes, or until each side is browned. Repeat until all patties are fried and drain on a paper towel. Each serving consists of 3 patties.

486 calories, 34.8 g fat, 37.8 g protein, 2.9 net carbs per serving

Makes 3 servings

HERRING

Herring may only be a mildly flavored medium-sized fish, but it doesn't lack nutrients despite its smaller size. It has945 mg of Omega-3 fatty acids, along with vitamin D, vitamin B12, and selenium. This type of fish has many serving options to fit your preference as well. You could eat it canned, fresh, served cold, precooked, and pickled. So many serving options give you a lot of opportunities for different recipes.

HERRING SALAD WITH BEETROOT

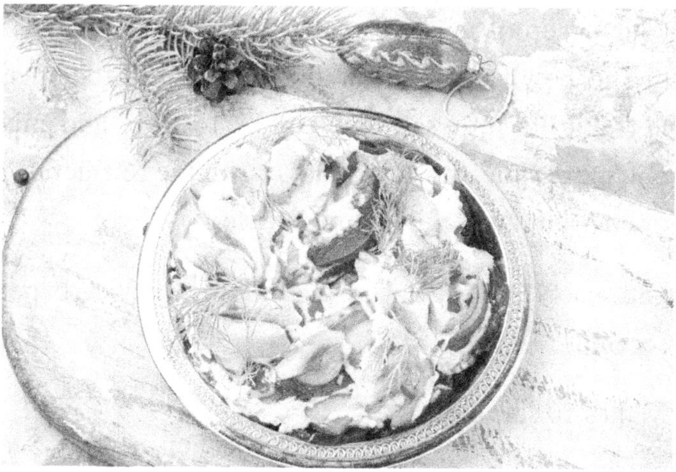

6 fillets (250 g) herring
3.5 oz (100 g) pickles slices, or 7 tablespoons pickle relish
3.5 oz (100 g) red onion, chopped
4 slices (50 g) pickled beetroot, chopped
½ cup (4 oz) sour cream, full fat
½ cup (4 oz) mayonnaise
salt and pepper, to taste

Cut the herring fillets into cubes. If you are using salted herring, be sure to soak the fillets in water for an hour before you cut them up. Chop up your pickles, if using slices, and mix them together with the chopped red onion and pickled beetroot in a small mixing bowl with the cubed herring fillets. Add in your ½ cup of sour cream and ½ cup of mayonnaise to the bowl and mix all the ingredients together. Sprinkle in your salt and pepper to taste and mix one more time. Store in a glass jar in the refrigerator or eat right away with some lettuce.

158 calories, 15 g fat, 4 g protein, 1 net carb per serving

Makes 10 servings

OYSTERS

Oysters are considered a delicacy, but those little clammed creatures have enough zinc, vitamin B12, omega-3's, and copper to meet your daily dietary needs. These delightful fishy treats can be enjoyed raw or cooked drizzled in butter.

KETO FRIED OYSTERS

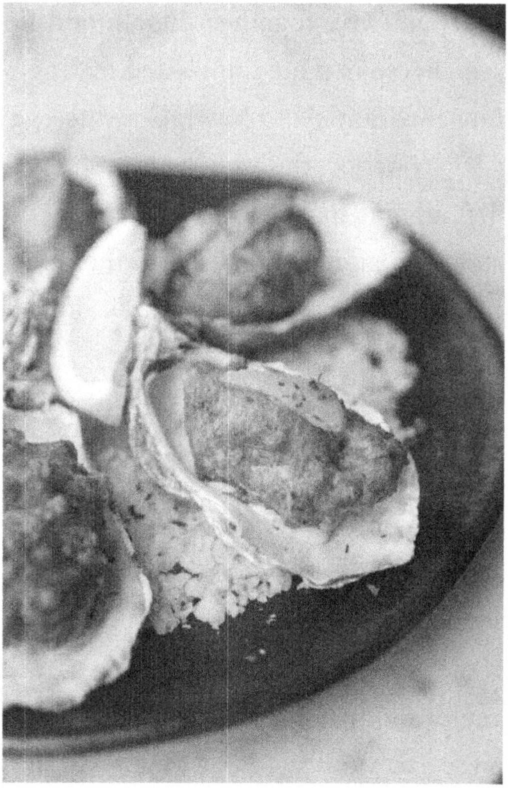

12 (about 3.5 oz) oysters, shucked
½ cup (48 g) almond flour
¼ cup (25 g) parmesan cheese, finely grated
1 large egg
salt, to taste
extra virgin olive oil or ghee, for frying

Shuck your oysters and place them on a paper towel. Pat them dry with another paper towel before you go any further. Mix together the almond flour and parmesan cheese in a medium-sized mixing bowl. In a separate medium-sized bowl, beat the egg with a whisk. Dip one of the shucked oysters into the almond flour and parmesan cheese mix, then into the beaten egg, and then back into the dry mix. Set aside on a clean paper towel until all of the oysters have been well-coated.

Heat your extra virgin olive oil or ghee in a frying pan over medium-high heat. Don't let the oil get too hot, though, you don't want the oysters coating to burn before the inside cooks. Place a few oysters into the oil once bubbles start to appear. Fry each side of the oysters until the coating is a golden-brown color, and transfer to a fresh paper towel to seep up the excess oil.

27 calories, 2 g fat, 1 gram protein, 0 carbs per oyster

Makes 12 oysters

TUNA

Canned tuna may be one of the most consumed fish in the United States, but fresh tuna has a different texture than one would expect. Fresh tuna has a denser but still satisfying flaky texture. Canned, fresh, and tuna steaks are full of other nutrients besides fatty acids, such as vitamin D, B12, and selenium just like the others.

AVOCADO TUNA MELT BITES

2 6.5-ounce canned tuna, drained
1 medium (201 g) avocado, cubed and pitted
¼ cup (59 g) parmesan cheese
¼ cup (2 oz) mayonnaise
⅓ cup (32 g) almond flour
½ cup (4 oz) coconut oil
½ teaspoon (1.5 g) garlic powder
¼ teaspoon onion powder
salt and pepper, to taste

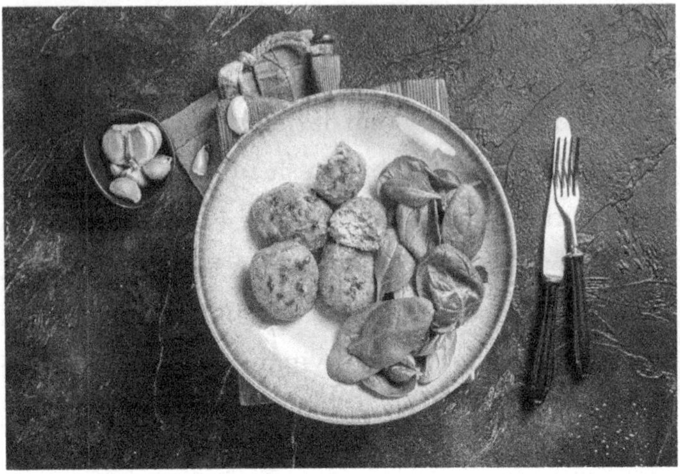

In a large mixing bowl, stir together the drained tuna, parmesan cheese, mayonnaise, and the spices. Remove the pit and slice the avocado into cubes while still in the skin so that the flesh isn't mashed. Carefully, fold the cubes of avocado into the tuna mixture. Use your hands to form the tuna-avocado mix into balls and roll the balls into the almond flour, covering the entire surface.

In a large frying pan, heat up the coconut oil over medium heat. Once the oil is hot and starting to bubble, place the tuna balls into the ball and fry until all sides are browned. Place the tuna bites onto a paper towel to soak up the extra oil.

185.2 calories, 17.8 g fat, 5 g protein, 1.02 net carbs per serving

Makes 12 servings (or bites)

SCALLOPS AND SHRIMP

These tender shellfish are low in fat and very high in protein. Both of them taste delicious with a creamy sauce or a drizzle of lemon juice over a bed of lettuce.

SCALLOPS IN GARLIC CREAM SAUCE

1 pound (454 g) of scallops, thawed
2 tablespoons (28.4 g) butter, unsalted
2 tablespoons (26.6 g) extra virgin olive oil
½ cup (4 oz) heavy whipping cream
¼ cup (2 oz) chicken broth
2 tablespoons (11.2 g) parmesan cheese, grated
1 tablespoon (5 g) garlic, minced
1 teaspoon (4.8 g) lemon juice
¼ teaspoon hot sauce
½ tablespoon dill, chopped if fresh
salt and pepper, to taste

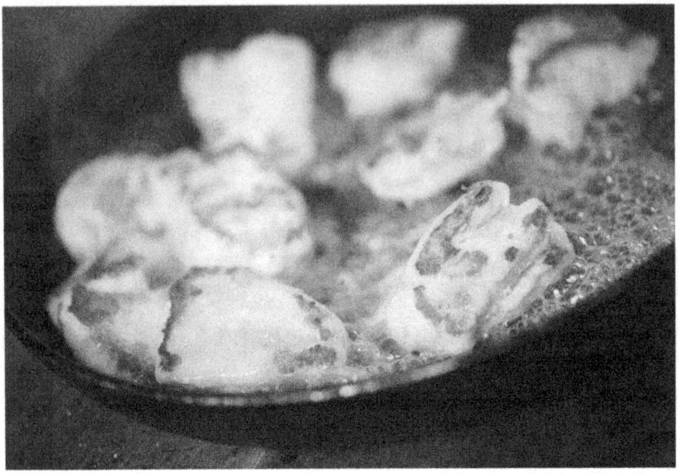

Rinse the thawed scallops in cold water and pat dry before seasoning them with the salt and pepper. Pour your olive oil into a frying pan and turn the heat to medium. Once the oil is hot, add the scallops to the pan and cook them for about 3 minutes per side. After all of the scallops are cooked, remove them from the frying pan and place aside so you can make the sauce.

In the same oil that you cooked the scallops in, add the butter and garlic to the frying pan and stir together, scraping all of the small bits left behind from the scallops. Add the chicken broth and lower the heat of the stove. Stir the sauce mixture occasionally for the next 5 minutes. Bring the heat down to a simmer and pour in the heavy whipping cream, parmesan cheese, hot sauce, and lemon juice. Let it simmer for about 8 to 10 minutes, stirring often to help the sauce thicken.

When the sauce is thickened to your preference, add the scallops back to the pan and mix them in with the sauce. Cover the pan after you sprinkle the fresh dill on top, and allow the entire meal to simmer for a few minutes. Serve immediately. You can eat this with spiralized veggies, zoodles, or over a bed of spinach.

349 calories, 26.5 g fat, 23.5 g protein, 8 net carbs

Makes 4 servings

SHRIMP AVOCADO SALAD

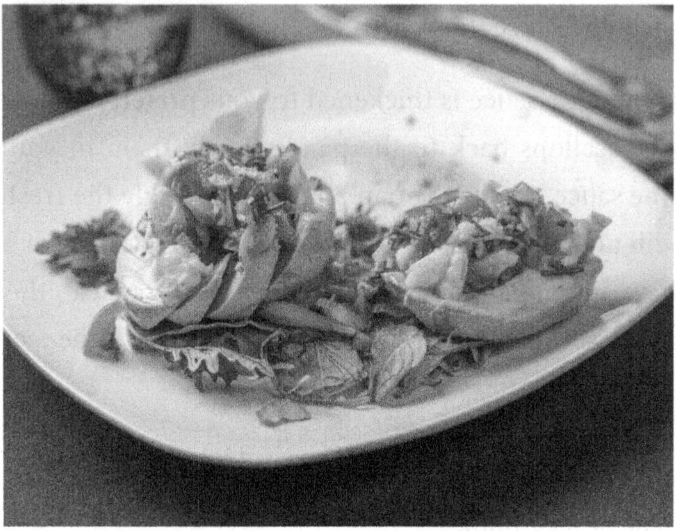

1 pound (454 g) raw shrimp, deveined and peeled

1 whole (201 g) avocado, diced and pitted

¼ cup (40 g) onion, chopped

1 whole (123 g) tomato, diced small

1 whole (14 g) jalapeno, minced and seeded (optional)

¼ cup (2 oz) lime or lemon juice, fresh

1 teaspoon (4.4 g) olive oil

1 tablespoon (6 g) coriander, chopped

salt and pepper, to taste

Cook the pound of raw shrimp in a frying pan with a small amount of olive oil, and chop into small pieces. In a large mixing bowl, mix the olive oil, fresh lemon or lime juice, salt, and pepper with a whisk. Toss in your avocado, red onion, shrimp, tomato, and cilantro into the bowl. You can add the jalapeno at this time as well if you choose to add one. Stir until the diced ingredients are completely covered in the sauce, cover with a lid and chill the meal until you are ready to serve.

240 calories, 10.5 g fat, 27.3 g protein, 5.6 net carbs per serving

Makes 4 servings

MAHI-MAHI

Mahi-mahi is a sweet, mild-flavored white fish that is low in fat, but makes up for it with 25 g of protein per serving. It contains the same vitamins as the other fish; however, it is much more versatile. It can be used as an alternative in any recipe that requires white fish.

MAHI-MAHI WITH WHITE WINE BUTTER SAUCE

6 3-ounce Mahi-mahi fillets
¼ pound (4 oz) bacon, raw
1 stick (8 tablespoons/113.6 g) butter, cut into ½ tablespoon portions
¼ cup (2 oz) extra virgin olive oil
¼ cup (2 oz) white wine
¼ cup (2 oz) heavy whipping cream
1 tablespoon (15 g) dill, chopped
2 tablespoons fresh parsley, chopped
lemon juice, fresh from 1 lemon
salt and pepper, to taste

Fry the strips of bacon on medium heat until crispy on both sides. Remove the bacon from the pan, chop them up, and put aside. Reserve the bacon grease for later. Heat the olive oil in the frying pan over a medium-high flame, and season your 3-ounce fillets with salt and pepper while the oil warms up.

Once the oil is hot and starting to bubble, sear one side of the fillet and flip 3 minutes later when the fish is cooked halfway through. Cook the other side until the fish fillet is cooked all the way through.

Remove the cooked fillets and put them on a plate, keeping the pan on the flame.

Add the ¼ cup of white wine and let the oil-wine mixture reduce until it becomes syrup-like. Pour in the heavy whipping cream and the reserved bacon grease that you set aside earlier, and remove the pan from the heat. Add the ½ tablespoon slices of butter and whisk in until they are completely melted and mixed into the sauce. Add the lemon juice, parsley, dill, chopped bacon, salt, and pepper and whisk them all together. Pour your sauce over the plated mahi-mahi fillets and enjoy!

360 calories, 30 g fat, 20 g protein, 1 net carb per serving

Makes 6 servings

BE IN CONTROL OF YOUR KETO DIET

The point is to be in control of your life and be in control of your keto diet. Choosing which plan works for you, whether it's the standard, cyclic, vegan, targeted, or high-protein plan, gives you a plethora of options. Only you can decide which option works best for you and makes you feel better.

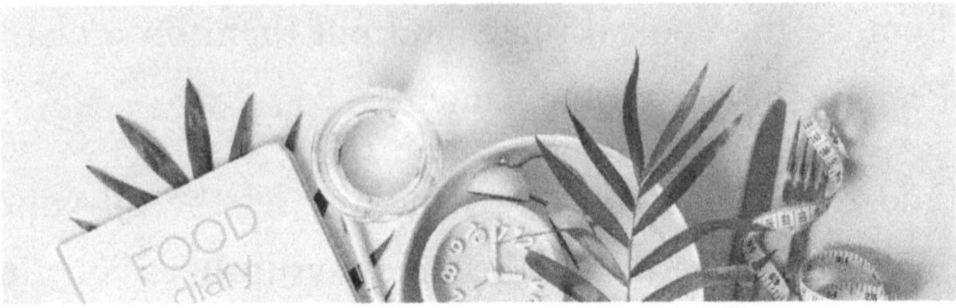

The best part about being in control of your diet is that once you learn how to make the meals and track them properly, you can start creating your own recipes. You will be aware of how many g in a serving of certain foods without having to look it up. You will know how many carbs are in each of your snacks and meals without having to research it. In other words, the adjustment period can be difficult, but it gets much easier with time.

8

DEBUNKING MYTHS AND FIXING COMMON MISTAKES

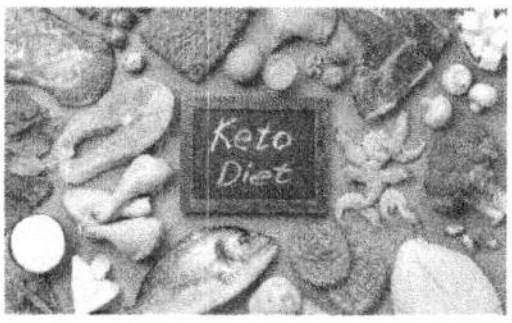

COMMON MISCONCEPTIONS OF THE KETO DIET

There is so much information available that it is hard to sort through what is fact and what is fiction when it comes to the keto diet. Many articles are written by people that are only stating what worked for them while some cite different medical studies. It can be confusing to new keto dieters.

- *A ketogenic diet is a new diet that is only used for weight loss.* The keto diet has been used since the early 1900s when it was first used to minimize seizures for epileptic children. Since then, keto has shown vast improvements in people dealing with Parkinson's Disease, heart disease, autism, hypoglycemia, cancer treatment, thyroid disorders, autoimmune disorders, diabetes, migraines, depression, and polycystic ovary syndrome.

- *You can eat as much bacon and cheese as you want.* While cheese and bacon are delicious, you can't just pile them up on a plate and eat as much as you want to. Remember that even though bacon and cheese are filled with protein and fats, they also contain calories. You need a caloric deficit to lose weight and eating a lot of these items can put you over your daily calorie goal. Bacon and cheese are also low on fiber, and consuming too much can cause stomach troubles, problems with digestion, and constipation.
- *Ketogenic diets are temporary and you can stop once you lose the weight.* A ketogenic diet is more than a diet—it's a lifestyle. After a few months of staying on a strict keto eating plan, you will be surprised to see that you don't miss those sugary and carb-filled foods

anymore. If you get a craving for something, you will figure out how to make it keto-friendly. A keto lifestyle has a great takeaway once you meet your weight goal: It's sustainable and it lowers the chances of other health problems.

- *Keto allows you to eat any kind of fat.* The keto diet may be a high-fat diet, but that doesn't mean any kind of fat is acceptable. The diet calls for healthy fats, such as avocados, extra virgin olive oil, and full-fat dressings. The healthy fats that you need to consume give you a feeling of fullness for longer amounts of time. However, eating too many fats can leave you feeling uncomfortable and sick.
- *Everyone needs to follow the same carb restrictions.* Since nobody loses weight the same, it makes sense that not everyone can get or stay in ketosis by consuming or restricting the same amount of carbs. While some keto dieters can manage to get into ketosis by keeping their carbohydrate intake around 50 net carbs per day, others find it difficult if they eat more than 20 net carbs a day, especially those with metabolism issues.

- *Fruits and vegetables are high in carbs and sugars, so you can't eat them on the keto diet.* Fresh produce is a source for carbohydrates, but they are also a source of vitamins, minerals, antioxidants, and fiber that your body needs to function effectively. Considering the fact that a common issue caused by eating a low-carb diet is constipation, you need to make sure that you are eating foods that are high in fiber. Some vegetables and fruits are considered to be high-carb; however, if you are consistent with your tracking, you could fit some in here and there that go along with your daily macros.
- *The keto diet is considered a high-protein diet.* While the keto diet is similar to the Atkins diet due to it being a low-carb diet, protein should be eaten in moderation on the keto diet. Remember that protein gets transferred into glucose, so if you eat too much protein, it could kick you out of ketosis.
- *Keto is the best and only way that people can lose weight and keep it off.* As I stated before, nobody loses weight the same way because everyone is different. Think of all the

different diets that you had to try to find success with keto. The same goes for others, they may not be able to do the keto diet due to health issues. Medical problems like genetic mutation MTHFR can get worse from the diet's high concentration in the B6 vitamin; and people that have pre-existing heart blockages may experience worse symptoms due to the diet's high fat content.

- *Keto isn't a sustainable way to live.* As long as you are willing to keep up with the maintenance, cooking, meal planning, and sticking to the guidelines, you should be fine. Motivation is the biggest factor for this diet, as without it, you are going to have a hard time keeping the weight off and sustaining the benefits that you earned.
- *You can't drink alcohol on a keto diet.* While it is highly advised to cut back on your alcohol consumption, having a drink on occasion is possible, even on a ketogenic diet. Alcohol is full of yeast and sugar so it is full of carbs; however, there are alcoholic beverages that are considered low-carb. Seltzers, light beer, and vodka range from zero to four net carbs and are considered to be safe if they are

consumed in moderation. However, keep in mind while you are drinking that you will become intoxicated a lot faster than you used to. Carbs, such as greasy food and breading, soak up alcohol and the lack of having them in your stomach can make you feel quite tipsy after a few drinks.

- *You can't go to restaurants or eat fast food on keto.* Once you know what you can eat and what you should avoid while on a ketogenic diet, eating outside of the home becomes less stressful. Many businesses acknowledge that there are people who don't eat carbs and accommodate their dietary restrictions. Five Guys Burgers and Fries, In and Out Burger, and some fast-food chains allow you to omit the buns and put the contents of your meal in a bowl for you to enjoy. You can request to leave off certain condiments, like ketchup, or have your dressing on the side so you can be in control of how much you use.

COMMON MISTAKES MADE BY KETO BEGINNERS

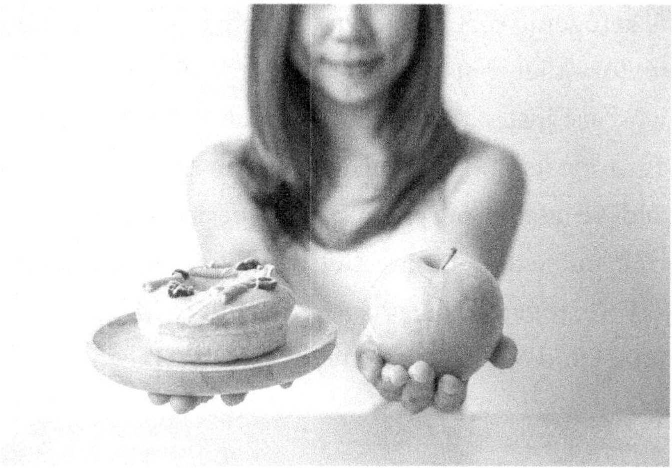

Just like the common misconceptions about the keto diet spread through the Internet like wildfire, so does misinformation. This misinformation is confusing to people just beginning their keto diet journey and leads to mistakes that can become detrimental to their progress if they aren't corrected. These common mistakes include:

EATING TOO MANY HIGHLY INFLAMMATORY FOODS

A ketogenic diet is known for being an anti-inflammatory diet, but it is not uncommon to see dieters who are just starting out fill up on processed, packaged meats and low-quality cooking oils. Slim Jims and vegetable oil are okay for occasional use, but lack nutrients and are full of fillers and trans fats. Try to replace the processed foods with grass-fed meats and oils, such as olive or coconut oil.

NOT EATING ENOUGH LOW-CARB VEGGIES

Vegetables are full of nutrients, vitamins, and fiber that your body desperately needs, especially once you cut out other groups of food. Veggies that grow above ground like zucchini, cucumbers, tomatoes, pumpkin, green beans, and spinach are all considered to be low-carb for a keto diet. However, starchy vegetables that have a high carb content, such as potatoes, squash, beans, peas, and corn, should be avoided as much as possible.

PUTTING TOO MUCH PRIORITY ON YOUR KETONE LEVELS, RATHER THAN HOW YOU FEEL

When you first start the keto diet, it's exciting to see your ketone levels rise. It means your hard work and willpower are paying off, although you should not expect them to keep rising the further along you go. In the beginning, the high ketone levels are a sign that your body isn't used to using ketones for a fuel source and you have more fat to burn, but the number will start to top off eventually. Try not to focus on the number on the scale. Instead, focus on inches lost, energy level, sleep quality, and your mood as an indicator of how you are doing.

INCLUDING TOO MUCH DAIRY INTO YOUR DIET

It's quite easy to go overboard with dairy. It's delicious, filling, high-fat, and makes food taste better. However, dairy comes with its own warning label on what it can do to you and your ketosis. Some people are unaware of their body's sensitivity to dairy products. They may not get sick, but a small allergy or sensitivity can wreak havoc on their digestion or cause varying degrees of inflammation. Dairy is also considered to be calorie-dense, so you may be eating more calories than you are burning if you don't keep an eye or measure how much you are consuming.

BECOMING TOO STRESSED

Believe it or not, changing how you eat can be considered a huge change in your life. A huge change or shift can create stress that you haven't dealt with before. However, be aware of what happens if you become too stressed out. When stress levels rise, so do cortisol levels. When cortisol levels rise, the body releases your stored glucose that causes your blood sugar to rise. A body that is in a constant state of stress, with overwhelming levels of cortisol in its system, is less resistant to the body's natural insulin and glucose is free to circulate around the bloodstream. It is highly recommended that during the beginning stages of keto that you abstain from making any other big changes in your life, like changing jobs or moving. If a high stress level has always been a problem for you, try finding ways to relieve your stress like yoga or deep meditation. After all, less stress equals more success.

RELYING ON SWEETENER ALTERNATIVES TOO OFTEN TO DEAL WITH YOUR SWEET TOOTH

Using artificial sweeteners like stevia, or ones that contain sucrose and aspartame, may not add carbs onto your daily intake, but they can cause a stall in your weight loss, inflammation, and digestive problems if you use them too often. Sugar lights up the same reward receptors as cocaine, and artificial sweeteners aren't any different. You can become addicted to these alternatives the same way that you do to sugar, only increasing your cravings and making it harder to stay on track. Drinking diet soda can even make sugar cravings worse. If that is the case, try switching out your zero-sugar soda with sparkling water.

CONSUMING TOO MANY LOW-CARB GRAINS

Finding a low-carb tortilla or zero-carb bread sounds like a dream after you haven't eaten either of those items for months, or in some cases years. However, keep in mind that these items do contain flour, grains, and carbs; they just have little to no net carbs thanks to the fiber. Having flour and carbs involved means that glucose will be introduced into your system, and consuming too much of the bread could kick you out of ketosis. If you find that you are stuck on a plateau, try cutting out any low-carb grains for a week and see if it makes a difference.

NOT EATING ENOUGH PROTEIN

During ketosis, a process called 'gluconeogenesis' occurs that helps your body to function by releasing small amounts of glucose. Glucose is considered to be bad for the keto diet, but the body still needs it to function properly. Gluconeogenesis helps stabilize blood sugar, prevent episodes of hypoglycemia, and assists the tissues that can't metabolize ketones. Eating the proper amount of protein can also aid in your weight loss by keeping you feeling fuller for extended amounts of time.

MAKING A DRASTIC CHANGE IN THEIR EATING HABITS TOO QUICKLY

The body does have the ability to adapt to anything; however, it is best to ease into the change rather than go cold turkey. Your body may not enjoy carbo-loading one day and then the next only ingesting 25 net carbs a day. It would go into a small state of shock, and guarantee the beginning of the dreaded 'keto flu.' Easing into a low-carb, high-fat lifestyle is easier than shocking your body into submission.

NOT PAYING ATTENTION TO HOW MANY VEGETABLES YOU ARE EATING

All vegetables contain carbohydrates, even the less threatening ones like lettuce. Eating them as much as possible may seem like a great idea, but if you aren't careful, you could do more harm than good. Vegetables are important as they contain micronutrients that you need, and fiber that can keep you from getting constipated. Just be sure to mind your portions and caloric intake.

FORGETTING TO ADD ENOUGH SALT TO THEIR FOOD

If you lived on processed foods for most of your life, people probably told you to watch your sodium levels. Now that you are on keto, you still need to watch it and add a little bit more. Strange, right? The reason is because now that you have cut out the processed, packaged food, like bread, chips, and bagels, you are actually consuming less salt. Your body could lose even more sodium if you become dehydrated. So don't be shy, shake that salt shaker!

NOT PLANNING AHEAD FOR THE KETO FLU

If you don't plan for the keto flu beforehand, you will feel like a semi-truck ran over you and backed over you twice. It is best to be prepared so you aren't down for the count for possibly seven days, if the symptoms aren't too severe. Making sure that you stay hydrated, consume enough electrolytes (especially salt), and pace yourself when cutting back on your carbs can minimize the symptoms even if you do get stuck with the keto flu.

FOCUSING ON QUANTITY OVER QUALITY IN REGARD TO FOOD

Sure a large plate of food sounds great when you are starving, but wouldn't you prefer a meal that leaves you feeling full for a long amount of time, rather than a large meal that only leaves you feeling full for an hour or so? Focusing on the quality of your food is much more important than the quantity. Meals that are dense in nutrients, vitamins, and healthy fats will give you a more satisfying energy boost and leave you feeling full longer than a large platter of empty calories. Nutrient-dense meals will also help you lose weight in the long run, considering that you will have less desire to snack throughout the day and lower your chances of being exposed to the keto flu.

HEAVY WHIPPING CREAM HAS CARBS, EVEN IF THE CONTAINER SAYS ZERO GRAMS

Heavy whipping cream is an awesome keto-friendly ingredient. It's full of fat, it makes your food creamy, and contains hidden carbs that add up through the day! Wait a minute, hidden carbs? Yes, a cup of heavy whipping cream contains 6.6 carbs even if the container reads zero carbs. While it is considered keto-friendly, it's best to keep in mind how much you are actually using because even small amounts add up throughout the day.

FORGETTING TO MEAL PLAN

After a year or so, meal planning becomes routine and starts to burn you out. But think about it, isn't your life much easier when you know what you are doing ahead of time? Isn't knowing what meals you plan to make, track, and buy ingredients for much more beneficial for your health than running through the drive-thru? Meal planning may not be a blast, but with this diet you get back what you put into it.

AN APPLE A DAY KEEPS KETOSIS AWAY

I'm sure as a young child you heard about the importance of eating apples. However, one small apple contains 20 net carbs! So, if you have managed to lower your carb allowance to 25 net carbs a day and you eat an apple with a serving of peanut butter, you have eaten all of your nets in one day.

NOT PAYING ATTENTION TO HIDDEN CARBS IN YOUR FOOD

Foods like salad dressing, zero-sugar sports drinks, and processed meats all have hidden carbs. Remembering to read the ingredients on the food label properly can ensure that you know exactly what you are eating and if any sugars are hiding in there. It is also helpful to know exactly what is in your food, especially at restaurants. If your server is unable to tell you exactly what is in your meal, ask them to put any sauces or dressings on the side.

NOT PAYING ATTENTION TO SERVING SIZES

On each nutrition label, there is a serving size. Some may say a particular measurement or weight, but it's very important to pay attention to the amount that the label reads. That is where a food scale comes in handy, so that you can make sure the serving that you are eating is on track with how much you calculated. Even foods that are marketed as low-carb or keto-friendly can be tricky. A keto cookie can read as 4 net carbs on the front but if you read the nutrition label, it is broken into two or three servings.

HOW TO STAY KETO WHEN YOU GET SICK

It's not a subject that many people think about on a daily basis. What happens if I get a cold or the flu? How will I eat my chicken noodle soup if I don't eat carbs? What medicine can I take? I'm sure that the last question hasn't occurred to you yet. Consider the fact that one dose of NyQuil has 20 net carbs per dose, and you have been successful in cutting your carb intake to 25 net carbs per day. By the time that you are ready to take your next dose, you will be on your second day's carb allowance from the fillers and sugar in the liquid medicine. However, if you take the pill form of the same medication, that is only 6 net carbs per dose. It may be more carbs than you planned, but it is a more viable option.

A keto diet can help you feel better quicker though! Following the same rules about hydration, electrolytes, and sticking to whole foods, like vegetables and proteins, can give your immune system the boost it needs while keeping you in ketosis. A few more things to try when you are fighting a sickness and keep yourself in a state of ketosis:

- Supplementing with bone broth between meals and adding lemon and ginger to your water can keep your electrolytes up while settling an upset stomach.
- Kick your fever and muscle pains by alternating ibuprofen and acetaminophen so you don't have to worry about extra carbs.
- Soothe your sore throat by adding oregano oil or Himalayan salt to a glass of warm water, gargle and spit out.

- Add electrolyte powder to your water bottles. Powerade and Gatorade Zero have many water-flavoring packets that not only taste great but will give you the electrolytes that you need so you don't become dehydrated.
- If you feel the need to indulge in some hearty soups to aid what ails you, check out the instant pot recipes in Chapter 4.

9

STAY MOTIVATED WITH KETO SUCCESS STORIES

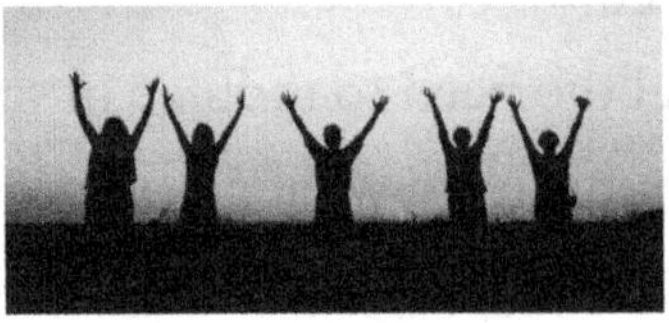

CAROLINE'S KETO SUCCESS STORY

Throughout her childhood and many of her teenage years, Caroline struggled with her weight. She was active in all sports, including soccer, volleyball, tennis, track, and running triathlons, but her weight kept going up and down. Her frustration with her weight caused her to focus on strength training in hopes that it would help her lose those stubborn pounds.

By her early twenties, Caroline weighed over 300 pounds and was still gaining, even though she was still very active. She was able to get down to 230 pounds after restricting her food intake severely and doing extreme resistance training for over 2 ½ hours a day. The weight loss was unsustainable and unhealthy, so when she went back to eating normally her weight started to go up again.

Within five years, she had only lost 18 pounds and had started to run out of options. Caroline knew that she needed to lose weight but wasn't sure where to turn or what to do. In the spring of 2017, she had to make a trip to the emergency room with complaints of an inflamed gallbladder. The medical provider who oversaw her treatment that night politely hinted that she should try losing weight.

Caroline made a follow-up appointment with her family doctor two days later, and her doctor told her that she should look into a ketogenic diet paired with intermittent fasting. If keto didn't work for her, the only option she would have left is an invasive surgical choice, like bariatric surgery. Caroline had researched bariatric surgeries before and knew about the complications and failure rates that often went along with the surgery. She decided to go ahead and give keto a try.

Within no time, Caroline had fine-tuned her personal keto ratios to what worked for her and was able to start losing weight by restricting her net carbs to 20 per day. In the first six weeks, she lost 28 pounds and was much happier since she didn't have to restrict her calorie intake and exercise for hours on end. Today, Caroline has lost over 80 pounds and is so proud of the progress she has made. She still works out and trains very hard, but can now afford to take a day off every once in a while.

CARI'S KETO SUCCESS STORY

After Cari's 40th birthday, she and her husband decided to make a life change and switch to a ketogenic lifestyle. She was tired of feeling like she was 60 and knew that she had to do something. Her sister had visited her from out of state for her birthday and had been on the keto diet for only a few months, losing a large amount of weight in that short amount of time. Her sister's progress blew her away and sparked the inspiration that she needed.

Cari's weight gain started when she lost her dad, mom, and stepdad to cancer within a few years of each other. They were all pretty young when they passed, all three in their mid-50s, and Cari took each loss harder than the last. She had stopped taking care of herself and was overcome with crippling grief. Within nine months, Cari's anxiety was so bad that she couldn't leave the house. But in the back of her mind, she knew that if she didn't start taking care of herself that her children may face the same reality as she was at that time. They could possibly lose their mother, and if she didn't do something about it, it would be her own fault.

She tracked her meals religiously, and she was strict with her clean-food choices. Cari didn't buy into prepackaged keto snacks, fat bombs, sweetened drinks, or desserts. She didn't even engage in cheat days or meals. She stayed on track, but chose not to use intermittent fasting to aid her in her weight loss. She kept her meals simple because she hates cooking, and she has never been much of a snacker.

Cari knows how stubborn she is but that strong-willed mentality is what helped her succeed. She never questioned herself or her commitment to getting healthier. Her willpower helped her fight off cravings for the first two weeks, and it was smooth sailing after that. Her energy level started to go up as her weight went down, and she was back to loving life again. Today, Cari is celebrating the loss of 100 pounds in under a year and is so happy to have her life back.

GAVIN'S LIFESAVING KETO SUCCESS STORY

By the time Gavin was three years old, he was having hundreds of seizures a day. They were considered drop seizures and would go on consistently throughout the day, occasionally causing him to drop to the ground. His first diagnosis had his parents believing that he would never be fully potty trained or go to school like a normal child.

Gavin's parents went from doctor to doctor, and then specialist to specialist for second, third, and fourth opinions. They finally met with a neurologist at their local children's hospital, where Gavin was diagnosed with Doose Syndrome. The neurologist suggested that Gavin's parents start him on a modified keto diet.

His diet was modified to only consume 10 carbs a day maximum, and his parents were so happy to see results within a few days. Gavin had stopped seizing almost instantly, and was able to be removed from his anti-seizure medications that had side effects almost as bad as the seizures themselves.

Gavin has been on the keto diet for five years now and has been seizure-free for the same amount of time. He is a straight-A middle-school boy that loves bacon and eggs. Sometimes he gets frustrated at birthday parties and when he's out with friends because he can't eat the same food that they can, but he finds a way to make it work. Gavin's parents are so thankful for his neurologist, medical advancement, and the keto diet. They know without those three things that their son wouldn't be thriving nearly as much as he is today.

ALVIN'S KETO SUCCESS STORY

Alvin was dealing with a lot of medical issues when he was 332 pounds. He was dealing with COPD, chronic pain, pre-diabetes, pulmonary hypertension, and metabolic syndrome. He was sick and exhausted all the time, and it seemed like no matter what he ate within an hour he would be hungry again. He was spiraling towards an early death, and his family doctor confirmed that within five years Alvin would be dead if he didn't change his ways.

He was aware of what a low-carb diet was, and it just didn't make any sense to him. Restriction carbs went against everything he learned in health class. Alvin had only learned that in order to lose weight, you have to cut down on your calories. When he tried to count his calories, he was never able to stick with it long term because he was always too hungry to stick with the plan. Alvin would cheat on his diet, overeat or eat what he wasn't supposed to, and then he would eat more because he felt guilty about it.

So he started doing his own research, and after reading up on the keto diet, he decided to try it for a month. The first week was the hardest for him. His cravings for potatoes, sweets, and bread grew stronger, but he stuck with it because he knew they would eventually pass. Alvin got the keto flu for a few days, with the exhaustion and muscle aches to boot. He felt like a drug addict going through withdrawal, but this passed as well. Once the keto flu passed, it was as if the clouds had parted and suddenly the fog was gone. He could think clearly and felt energy like he never had before. His food cravings also disappeared with his exhaustion and cravings.

He was surprised that once he ate until he felt full first thing in the morning, he could make it through a majority of the day with a handful of nuts and some deviled eggs. Then, for dinner, he could have a large slab of meat with a salad and be set for the day. After nine months, Alvin was down 56 pounds, but life ended up getting in the way. He went back to eating all of the foods that he had given up and regained 25 pounds.

Once he was wavering over the 300-pound mark, and he was back to being sick, tired, and miserable again. Alvin had started to give up on losing weight, until his girlfriend agreed to do the keto diet with him. He lost the weight that he had gained back and 40 more pounds over the next six months, and his girlfriend wasn't far behind him, losing six dress sizes in that time. They intend on cutting back to consuming less than 15 net carbs a day once they get close to their goal weight to carry them over the finish line.

ELEANORE'S KETO SUCCESS STORY

Throughout Eleanore's entire life, she struggled with her weight. Being born without a thyroid left her with a small, almost non-existent, metabolism. She managed to stay thin through her teenage years, but became obsessed with the possibility of becoming obese as she got older. She participated in unhealthy eating habits, like binging and purging, starving herself, and diet pills to keep herself thin but only ended up feeling more depressed and more obsessed with what the future held.

Eleanore wasn't a stranger to toxic relationships, and after an abusive three-year relationship left her pregnant and alone, she had to deal with a newborn baby and postpartum depression on her own. By the age of 23, she had given birth to two more children with a man she married two years after the birth of her first child. Her depression got worse after each child, and so did the constant eating. Her doctor put her on psychiatric medications that only made her gain more weight, or put her in a manic state. She managed to lose weight once when she was 25, but did it in unhealthy ways. Eleanor would work out three hours a day and cut her calories below 1,000 a day to ensure that she burned everything that she ate. She was proud to go from 230 pounds to 190 in a matter of three months, but that weight loss and diet plan were not sustainable.

Eleanore gained the weight back, and by the time she was 30, she weighed almost 300 pounds. She only stood 5'3," so the excess weight was very noticeable. She felt sick and exhausted all the time, grouchy and short-tempered with her family, and felt sad that she never had the energy to play with her children. Plus, the costs of her constant lab work, specialist visits, and dosage increases in her thyroid medication were really starting to add up. In February 2018, she started to feel sharp chest pains and her husband took her to the emergency room. The doctor told her that she didn't have a heart attack, but she should consider losing weight or she may not be so lucky next time.

She kept the doctor's words in the back of her mind for a few months, as she tried to ignore the symptoms of her body fighting her with every step. It got to the point that she couldn't walk across the room without being out of breath and sweating, and the extra weight was making her body go into early menopause.

By August 2018, she couldn't deal with her weight anymore, and her husband agreed to go on the keto diet with her. She did all of the research, uploaded the apps, and bought everything she needed to start.

The weight fell off quickly. Within a month, she had lost 25 pounds eating food she loved and felt great. She introduced the 16:8 intermittent fasting plan to her schedule, and began walking the park every morning after she dropped her kids off at school.

The exercise helped with her weight loss but she had to take a two-hour nap afterward.

By two months, Eleanore had lost 40 pounds and had started running six miles every morning. She no longer felt tired after exercising, and had enough energy to go through the day without slowing down. She made it her goal to run a 5k within the next year, something she had made fun of other people for doing when she was overweight. She didn't care about her placement though, she just wanted to be able to do it.

Her plans hit a snag after being on the keto diet for five months when she was rear-ended and broke her leg. She had to do six months of physical therapy three times a week, but still managed to lose 50 pounds while on crutches because she followed a strict keto plan to make up for her inability to exercise. Getting back to her walking schedule was harder than she thought after she was done with physical therapy. It was cold outside and her leg wasn't as strong as it was before the accident, but a few months later she was back to normal as long as she wore her knee brace.

Within a year and a half, Eleanore had met her goal weight a few times, kept going and pushed for a new goal. In the end, she had lost 135 pounds, which was literally half of her body weight before she started keto. She went from 4X sized clothes to wearing XX-Small, and even shares clothes with her teenage daughter. She has energy to play with her kids and kick the soccer ball around with her middle daughter. She went from being angry all the time to having a very calm and zen demeanor, using meditation when she is stressed out. She even started helping others start the keto journey by showing them how to track their food, making meal plans, and sharing her favorite recipes.

Eleanore did meet her goal of running a 5k in the fall of 2019, placing 7th in the nation and 5th in the women's bracket. She has been maintaining her weight loss for over a year now. Her husband did just as well as she did, losing over 130 pounds in 18 months. The couple found it so much easier to lose weight together, because they could hold each other accountable. Plus, Eleanore refused to make two dinners so he had no choice but to stay on track.

CREATE AND BECOME YOUR OWN KETO SUCCESS STORY

I hope that reading how other people overcame their addiction to processed food, sugar, and carbohydrates inspires you to create your own keto success story. You don't have to write it down or brag about it online—unless that is what you want to do. Some people do feel the need to show off their success in hopes of inspiring others to get healthy, but some prefer to celebrate their progress in private. Sometimes it is helpful when you feel like you are stuck to remember why you started the keto diet in the first place, or where you started versus where you are now.

Think about what happened that got you to the point that you knew you needed to change your life. Did a doctor tell you that you were at risk of losing your life or developing a life altering disease if you didn't lose weight? Were you becoming sick and tired of being sick and tired? Did you get embarrassed when you couldn't ride on a rollercoaster with your child because you were too big for the safety harness? Did you get an error message on the bathroom scale because it could no longer register your weight?

Everyone has an event or a feeling that sparked some inspiration to change their life and motivate them to stick with the plan. Even if they have tried and failed at multiple dietary restrictions and plans, eventually one may stick, just like the success stories that you just read.

All of the success stories did mention one similar feature: the cravings for the first week were the hardest part but the people chose to stick with it. Their motivation and willpower to lose weight was stronger than their cravings; all of them were afraid to lose their life because they couldn't stop eating unhealthy food. Some of them were terrified that their children would lose their parent because they couldn't get their life under control.

After you figure out what got you to the starting line, remember how hard you worked to lose the weight. Remember the willpower that it required to turn down that donut your coworker offered you, even though it smelled amazing. Remember how hard it was to walk away when your children have leftovers of your former favorite food, but you still did it.

You were able to stay motivated because you could see the big picture. You could see that finish line at the end of what you hoped to look like, feel like, and how much healthier you would be when this was all over. You focused on the fact that you may no longer need to take medication for your type II diabetes or high blood pressure if you lose the weight.

If you are almost at the finish line and at your goal weight, think about how much better you feel:

- What are your non-scale victories so far?
- Are you sleeping peacefully through the night without snoring?
- Can you walk up and down the stairs without being out of breath and needing to sit down to rest afterward?
- How many pant sizes have you gone down so far?
- How many inches have you shaved off of your entire body?
- Do you feel confident about yourself and what you see in the mirror?
- How is your mental health and do you feel much happier than you used to?

I know it seems like a lot of questions, but to see how successful your journey has been so far, you have to remember and acknowledge all of the changes and emotions that you went through to get you here.

Your story may not seem impressive to you, but there is someone out there who is watching how it all goes and becoming inspired with every pound you lost. Maybe it's your spouse, coworker, parent, or child. If you inspire someone that you care for and love to change their life and live healthier, wouldn't you want to make sure that your success story didn't end abruptly but with a celebration and new appreciation for life? How you write your keto success story is up to you, but make sure that it's inspiring, even if it only inspires you.

AFTERWORD

Knowing how a ketogenic lifestyle benefits you, your health, and your body can change your life. Becoming aware of what you eat, how much you eat, and how to track your meals properly can transform your struggling body into a well-oiled, fat-burning machine.

How you go about your diet is all up to you. Whether you are a beginner or have been on the ketogenic diet for a while now, there is always room for improvement and updated information to learn. There is no longer a need to give up or get burnt out because of boring, bland food thanks to new and tasty alternatives. You could try a different keto plan or move onto a plant-based ketogenic lifestyle for a short time if you get tired of red meat. You can add new and effective workouts and exercises to your day that are tailored to you, your schedule, and your needs.

The one thing that I hope you take away from this book is that the only way to ensure that you are successful and able to sustain a keto lifestyle depends on your level of motivation. If you aren't motivated to stay on track, plan your meals, and completely change how you live your life, then you will have a harder time losing weight and maintaining any weight you have lost.

As long as you are prepared to make a complete change, then is your body. I can only give you the tools to guide you along the way.

If you enjoyed reading this book and gaining more insight on the keto diet, feel free to leave a review on Amazon.

REFERENCES

Alonso, M. (2020). *plank*. In Pexels. https://www.pexels.com/photo/active-asian-woman-doing-plank-at-home-7592988/

Alvin. (2014, June 13). *Success Stories: Alvin Fights Back with a Low Carb Diet*. No Bun Please. https://nobunplease.com/success-stories-alvins-fights-back-low-carb-diet/

Angela. (2019, December 4). *Keto Success Story: Cari Lost 100 Pounds & Got Her Life Back*. Hip2Keto. https://hip2keto.-com/tips/keto-success-story-cari-lost-100-pounds-life-back/

Baum, I. (2020). *Transform Your Abs With This At-Home Routine -* Perfect Keto. Perfectketo.com. https://perfectketo.com/ab-workout-routine/

Better Health Channel. (2012). *Walking for good health*. Vic.gov-.au. https://www.betterhealth.vic.gov.au/health/healthyliving/walking-for-good-health

Bond, D. (2020, July 5). *Easy Keto Mackerel Patties* | KetoDiet Blog. KetoDiet. https://ketodietapp.com/Blog/lchf/easy-keto-mackerel-patties#preptime

Bourdua-Roy, E. (2018, February 4). *"I had been trying to lose weight since the age of 9. And they told me all that I had left was bariatric surgery."* Diet Doctor. https://www.dietdoctor.-com/trying-lose-weight-since-age-9-told-left-bariatric-surgery

Brehm, B. J., Seeley, R. J., Daniels, S. R., & D'Alessio, D. A. (2003). *A Randomized Trial Comparing a Very Low Carbohydrate Diet and a Calorie-Restricted Low Fat Diet on Body Weight and Cardiovascular Risk Factors in Healthy Women*. The Journal of

Clinical Endocrinology & Metabolism, 88(4), 1617–1623. https://doi.org/10.1210/jc.2002-021480

Carter, E. (2020, May 18). *Keto Guacamole.* Pure and Simple Nourishment. https://www.pureandsimplenourishment.-com/keto-guacamole/

Ciccarelli, D. (2020, January 23). *14 Foods With Hidden Sugars* —Perfect Keto. Perfectketo.com. https://perfectketo.-com/hidden-sugars/

Ciccarelli, L. (2021, October 24). *10 Foods to Fight Your Sugar Cravings*—Perfect Keto. Perfectketo.com. https://perfectke-to.com/sugar-craving/

City Fish Market. (2020). *Where Can I Find The Best Seafood To Eat During A Keto Diet? City Fish Market Blog.* https://cfishct.-com/blog/best-seafood-to-eat-on-a-keto-diet/

Cleveland Clinic. (2020, October 6). *Ketogenic Diet For Epilepsy / Seizures.* Cleveland Clinic. https://my.clevelandclin-ic.org/health/treatments/7156-ketogenic-diet-keto-diet-for-epilepsy#:~:text=The%20ketogenic%20diet%20has%20been

Diana. (2020, February 8). *Air Fryer Chicken Fajitas. Little Sunny Kitchen.* https://littlesunnykitchen.com/air-fryer-chicken-fajitas/

Dolan, M. (2019, June 17). *What the Keto Diet Will Do to Your Workout.* EverydayHealth.com. https://www.everydayhealth.-com/fitness/what-keto-diet-will-your-workout/

Ede, G. (2019, June 30). *8 Reasons to Try Low-Carb for Mental Health.* Psychology Today. https://www.psychologytoday.-com/us/blog/diagnosis-diet/201906/8-reasons-try-low-carb-mental-health

Emily. (2019, December 4). *Keto Success Story: Cari Lost 100 Pounds & Got Her Life Back.* Hip2Keto. https://hip2keto.-com/tips/keto-success-story-cari-lost-100-pounds-life-back/

Exercise Bike. (2015, June 4). *8 Key Benefits of Exercise Bikes.*

ExerciseBike. https://www.exercisebike.net/blog/exercise-bike-benefits/

F-Bomb. (2020, June 29). *Mahi-Mahi with White Wine Butter Sauce {Keto, Low-Carb}*. FBOMB. https://www.dropanfbomb.-com/blogs/recipes/mahi-mahi-white-wine-butter-sauce

Freitas, V. (2021). *Person holding barbell.* In Pexels.

Georgina. (2017, February 23). *Low Carb Ratatouille*. Step Away from the Carbs. https://stepawayfromthecarbs.com/low-carb-ratatouille/

Gerri. (2021, January 31). *Zoodles with Avocado Sauce Recipe - So Easy, So Tasty & Keto Friendly!* My Keto Kitchen. https://www.myketokitchen.com/keto-recipes/keto-zoodles-avocado-sauce/

Gunnars, K. (2018, November 20). *10 Health Benefits of Low-Carb and Ketogenic Diets.* Healthline. https://www.healthline.-com/nutrition/10-benefits-of-low-carb-ketogenic-diets#Food-Fix:-Keto-Basics

Hecht, M. (2018). *Ketosis vs. Ketoacidosis: What's the Difference?* Healthline. https://www.healthline.com/health/ketosis-vs-ketoacidosis

Hikichi, T. (2018, October 15). *Avoid! Top Ketogenic Diet Myths and Mistakes That Will Ruin Your Results.* Health & Wellness Promoter. https://healthandwellnesspromoter.com/keto-genic-diet-myths-and-mistakes/

Hubbard, K. (2021, September 15). *The Pandemic Has Worsened the U.S. Obesity Epidemic*. U.S. News. https://www.usnews.-com/news/best-states/articles/2021-09-15/the-pandemic-has-worsened-americas-obesity-epidemic-report-finds

Hullett, A. (2021, October 29). *Kettlebell Swing Benefits Make It the Ultimate All-in-One Workout.* Greatist. https://greatist.com/fitness/benefits-of-kettlebell-swings

Intermountain Healthcare. (2017, November 2). *Beware the Keto Flu.* Intermountainhealthcare.org. https://intermountainhealthcare.org/blogs/topics/live-well/2018/03/beware-the-keto-flu/

Keto Living. (2015, July 2). *Avocado Tuna Melt Bites.* Ruled Me. https://www.ruled.me/avocado-tuna-melt-bites/

Ketogains. (2015, September 15). *Ketogains Ultimate Novice* Kettlebell/Dumbell Workout. Ketogains. https://www.keto-gains.com/2015/09/ketogains-novice-strength-training-program-5x5/

Ketologic. (2020). *The Keto Diet and Gut Health: How a Ketogenic Lifestyle Impacts Digestive Health.* KetoLogic. https://ketolog-ic.com/blogs/articles/keto-diet-gut-health

Konscious. (2018, June 4). *Keto Cardio That Supports Weight Loss.* Konscious Keto. https://konsciousketo.-com/blogs/keto/keto-cardio

Krug, T. (2019, September 6). *Scallops in Garlic Cream Sauce* {Low Carb | Keto | GF}. Trina Krug. https://trinakrug.com/scal-lops-in-garlic-cream-sauce/

Kubala, J. (2018, June 28). *The 9 Best Keto Supplements.* Healthline. https://www.healthline.com/nutrition/best-keto-supple-ments#TOC_TITLE_HDR_2

Larbi, M. (2020, December 7). *Vegan Keto Diet: Is It Possible? And What Are The Benefits?* Plant Based News. https://plantbased-news.org/lifestyle/vegan-keto-diet-possible-benefits/

Lawler, M. (2019, June 27). *5 Reasons It's Harder to Lose Weight With Age and What to Do About It* | Everyday Health. Everyday-Health.com. https://www.everydayhealth.-com/weight/weight-gain-and-aging.aspx

Lindberg, S. (2019, June 21). *Elliptical Benefits: 10 Reasons to Use This Cardio Machine.* Healthline. https://www.healthline.-com/health/fitness-exercise/elliptical-benefits#benefits

Link, R. (2020, March 17). *Working Out on Keto: All You Need to Know.* Healthline. https://www.healthline.com/nutri-tion/working-out-on-keto#best-exercises-for-keto

Link, R. (2020, March 18). *Keto Fruit: 9 Healthy Options.* Healthline. https://www.healthline.com/nutrition/keto-fruit

Livermore, S., & Flager, M. (2020, July 16). *Easy Keto Recipes for Vegans,* From Fritters to Waffles. Delish. https://www.delish.-com/cooking/g4837/vegan-keto-recipes/

Long, K., & Austin, K. (2020, February 17). *Debunking Common Keto Myths.* Clean Keto Lifestyle. https://cleanketolifestyle.-com/debunking-common-myths-around-keto/

lowcarbnocarb. (2018, May 23). *Keto Avocado Popsicles the MUST for summer days.* Low Carb No Carb. https://www.lowcarb-nocarb.com/keto-avocado-popsicles/

Mac, L. (2021, February 22). *Top 13 Common Keto Mistakes And How To Fix Them* - Perfect Keto. Perfectketo.com. https://perfectketo.com/keto-mistakes/

Malone, C. (2018, December 11). *The Whoosh Effect: Myth or Reality.* Ketogenic.com. https://ketogenic.com/the-whoosh-effect-myth-or-reality/

Manager, C. (2020). *The Complete Guide to Exercise & Keto. Carb Manager.* https://www.carbmanager.com/article/x1lc7x-eaaceaxwz3/the-complete-guide-to-exercise-and-keto/

Marita & Mattis. (2020, March 12). *Easy Herring Salad with Beetroot (Low Carb and Keto).* Love of Avocados. https://loveofav-ocados.com/easy-herring-salad-with-beetroot-low-carb-and-keto/#wpzoom-recipe-card

Maurois, A. (2018, March 9). *The Ups and Downs of Weight Loss: Why You Shouldn't Give Up.* Thriveglobal.com. https://thrive-global.com/stories/the-ups-and-downs-of-weight-loss-why-you-shouldn-t-give-up/

Metcalf, T. (2017, September 15). *Keto Fried Oysters Recip*e - [Low Carb, Gluten Free]. KETOGASM. https://ketogasm.-com/keto-fried-oysters-recipe-low-carb-gluten-free/

Migala, J. (2019a, January 7). *7 Keto Diet Myths You Shouldn't Believe.* EverydayHealth.com. https://www.everydayhealth.-

com/ketogenic-diet/diet/keto-diet-myths-you-shouldnt-believe/

Migala, J. (2019b, January 7). *8 Keto Diet Mistakes Beginners Should Avoid.* EverydayHealth.com. https://www.everydayhealth.-com/ketogenic-diet/diet/common-keto-mistakes-you-may-make-avoid-them/

Migala, J. (2019c, January 29). *Intermittent Fasting Keto: How It Works, Benefits, Risks, More* | Everyday Health. EverydayHealth.-com. https://www.everydayhealth.com/ketogenic-diet/intermittent-fasting-keto-how-it-works-benefits-risks-more/

My Budget Recipes. (2021). *Is An Air Fryer Good for Keto?* – My Budget Recipes. My Budget Recipes. https://mybudgetrecipes.com/is-an-air-fryer-good-for-keto/

Nast, C. (2017, June 8). *14 Beginner Kettlebell Exercises That Work Your Entire Body.* SELF. https://www.self.com/gallery/beginner-kettlebell-moves

Occhipinti, M. (2018). *What is the History and Evolution of the Keto Diet?* Afpafitness.com. https://www.afpafitness.-com/blog/what-is-the-history-and-evolution-of-the-keto-diet

Olsson, E. (2021). *Vegetable salad.* In Pexels. https://www.pexels.-com/photo/photo-of-vegetable-salad-in-bowls-1640770/

Petrovska, K. (2019, January 16). *Instant Pot Crack Chicken* | The Most Amazing Chicken Dinner. Diethood. https://diethood.-com/instant-pot-crack-chicken-recipe/

Pitre, U. (2020, June 17). *Instant Pot Low Carb Italian Sausage Kale Soup.* TwoSleevers. https://twosleevers.com/low-carb-italian-sausage-kale-soup/

Pixabay. (2021). *blue measuring tape.* In Pexels. https://www.pexels.com/photo/blue-tape-measuring-on-clear-glass-square-weighing-scale-53404/

Rodnae productions. (2021). *jump rope.* In Pexels.

https://www.pexels.com/photo/man-in-black-shirt-training-with-jumping-rope-7187927/

SCL Health. (2018). *What Are Macros And Why Should I Be Counting Them?* Www.sclhealth.org. https://www.sclhealth.org/blog/2018/10/what-are-macros-and-why-should-i-be-counting-them/

Shreiner, A. B., Kao, J. Y., & Young, V. B. (2015). T*he gut microbiome in health and in disease*. Current Opinion in Gastroenterology, 31(1), 69–75. https://doi.org/10.1097/mog.0000000000000139

Sisson, M. (2018, December 7). *Got "keto burnout"? Here's how to get back on the wagon*. Bodyandsoulau. https://www.bodyandsoul.com.au/diet/got-keto-burnout-heres-how-to-get-back-on-the-wagon/news-story/db362e1d5de5ec4c859656e0885464c2

Sun, L. (2021). *Woman Doing Yoga*. In Pexels. https://www.pexels.com/photo/photo-of-woman-doing-yoga-2294354/

thatlowcarblife. (2019, June 13). *Garlic Butter Salmon and Asparagus*. That Low Carb Life. https://thatlowcarblife.com/garlic-butter-salmon-and-asparagus/

Unsplash. (2018). Photo by Dana DeVolk on Unsplash. In unsplash.com. https://unsplash.com/photos/-Cb-dhW7tqg

Unsplash. (2019). Photo by Heather Ford on Unsplash. In unsplash.com. https://unsplash.com/photos/Ug7kk0kThLk

Unsplash. (2020). Photo by Total Shape on Unsplash. In unsplash.com. https://unsplash.com/photos/W2QVimqre4w

Unsplash. (2021). Photo by RUSLAN BOGDANOV on Unsplash. In unsplash.com. https://unsplash.com/photos/MceegunFZ9o

VanItallie, T. B., Nonas, C., Di Rocco, A., Boyar, K., Hyams, K., & Heymsfield, S. B. (2005). *Treatment of Parkinson's disease with diet-induced hyperketonemia: A feasibility study*. Neurology,

64(4), 728–730. https://doi.org/10.1212/01.wnl.0000152046.11390.45

Vogel, L. (2019, January 21). *How to Stay Keto When You're Sick.* Healthful Pursuit. https://www.healthfulpursuit.-com/2019/01/res-keto-when-sick/

Wade, B. (2016, May 27). *Discover the fitness benefits of aqua aerobics.* Just Swim. https://www.swimming.org/justswim/aqua-aerobics-benefits-equipment/

Made in the USA
Monee, IL
04 November 2026

67385562R00105